Men's Fit Kitchen

Dedication

I would like to dedicate this book to my beautiful mother who sadly passed away this year. You have always been a tower of strength and a great inspiration to me. I will miss you so much.

The contents of this book were carefully researched. However, all information is supplied without liability. Neither the author nor the publisher will be liable for possible disadvantages or damages resulting from this book.

Please note: For reasons of readability this book is written in the male speech form. Any references to trainers and participants of course include men and women.

Men's
Fit Kitchen
Your Guide to Fitness and Food

Meyer & Meyer Sport

British Library Cataloguing in Publication Data
A catalogue record for this book is available from the British Library

Men´s Fit Kichen

Maidenhead: Meyer & Meyer Sport (UK) Ltd., 2016
ISBN: 978-1-78255-070-9

All rights reserved, especially the right to copy and distribute, including the translation rights. No part of this work may be reproduced—including by photocopy, microfilm or any other means— processed, stored electronically, copied or distributed in any form whatsoever without the written permission of the publisher.

© 2015 by Meyer & Meyer Sport (UK) Ltd.
Aachen, Auckland, Beirut, Cairo, Cape Town, Dubai, Hägendorf, Hong Kong,
Indianapolis, Manila, New Delhi, Singapore, Sydney, Tehran, Vienna
 Member of the World Sport Publishers' Association (WSPA)
Manufacturing: Print Consult GmbH, München
ISBN: 978-1-78255-070-9
E-Mail: info@m-m-sports.com
www.m-m-sports.com

TABLE OF CONTENTS

Introduction 12

1   Alcohol 14

2   Water 16

3   Top Fat-Burning Foods 18

4   Processed Foods 20

5   Sugar 22

6   Nutrition 24
      Carbohydrates 27
      Fats 28
      Fibre 29
      Vegetables 29
      Fruits 30
      Nuts and Seeds 30
      Herbs 31

7   Breakfast 34
      Energy-Boosting Breakfast 36
      Honey, Nuts and Yoghurt 38
      Power Porridge 39
      Sweet Potato Hash 41
      Open-Faced Breakfast Club Sandwich 42
      Ingredients 42
      Eggs 44
      Power Protein Omelette 46

Egg and Asparagus 47
Almond Porridge 48
Open-Faced Peanut Butter Crunch 49
Protein Punch 50
Banana Pancakes 51
Salmon-Wrapped Asparagus 52

8 Lunch 54

Tuna and Bean Salad 57
Open-Faced Grilled Halloumi Sandwich 58
Summer Salad 59
Roasted Red Pepper and Tomato Soup 60
Pea and Rocket Soup 62
Chicken and Apple Salad 63
Tuna Boat 64
Tomato and Mozzarella Stack 65
Open-Faced Chicken Pitta 67
Tomato and Nectarine Salad 68
Zucchini Pasta 71
Grilled Halloumi and Asparagus 72
Tortilla Wrap 73

9 Dinner 74

Basil and Avocado Pasta 77
Cod with Coconut and Dill 78
Tuna and Bean Salsa 81
Salmon Cake 85
Crab Linguine 86
Scallops and Sweet Potato Fries 89
Cod With Baked Cherry Tomatoes 90
Baked Salmon With Quinoa 93
Beef Stir-Fry 94

Lemon Chicken	95
Chicken With Rice Noodles	96
Steak With Twin Mash	99

10 Light Bites 100

Double Stack Protein	102
Power Fries and Protein Dip	103
Zucchini Pizza Bites	104
Calamari and Bean Salad	105
Mixed Greens	106
Grilled Peaches	108
Bliss Balls	109
Minted Peas	111
Light Snack	112
Open-Faced Avocado Sandwich	113
Sweet Potato Crisps	114

11 Smoothies 118

Green Monster	119
Cardio Crush	120
Immune Booster Shot	120
Beta Blaster	121
Lean and Green Shot	121
Chilli Shot	122
Berry Booster	122

12 Running and Getting Started 124

Making Running Easy	124
What You Need to Get Started	125
Training Kit	126
Beating the Boredom	127
Warm Up, Cool Down and Stretch	129
Power Walking	133

Men´s Fit Kitchen

    Before You Start 136
    Your First Run 140

13 Exercise **154**

14 The Ultimate Outdoor Workouts **164**
    How to Get Stronger With a Log 165
    The Sandbag Workout 173
    The Stair Workout 179
    The Outdoor Workout 184

15 Repairing Your Body **194**

16 Keep Up the Good Work **202**

17 Acknowledgments **204**

    Credits 206

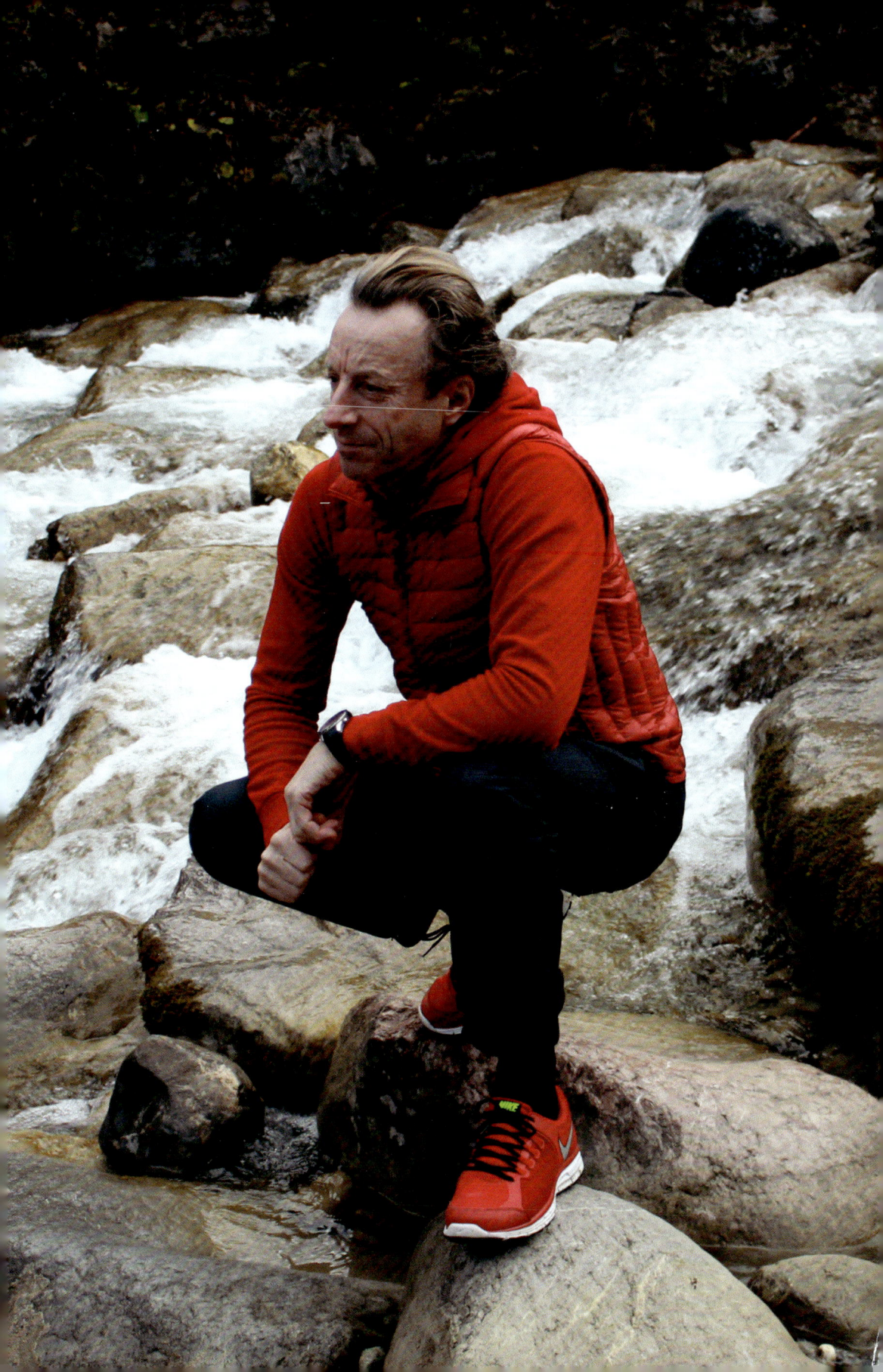

INTRODUCTION

Welcome to Men's Fit Kitchen!

In this book I will show you how easy it is to become a stronger and better man, and more importantly, a better version of yourself. I will show you how easy it is to make some mouth-watering recipes, easy and healthy snacks and powerful smoothies which will help you to lose weight and build muscle.

I will introduce you to some quick indoor and unique outdoor workouts which will help you burn fat and tighten up your body. I will also give you a complete beginner's running plan that covers all aspects of how to enjoy running. This running plan will get you started on the road to the new you.

A lot of men don't have time for arduous recipes that are time consuming and hard to follow. Meals that are simple to make, have easy instructions, and use high-quality ingredients and fresh fruits and vegetables will help you create a strong, lean and healthy body.

Like most of us, I have a very busy lifestyle, and food was never important to me. It was just a case of grab and go, and many nights involved takeaways, ready meals and beer. After years of feeling tired, lacking motivation and feeling bloated and generally very unhappy with myself, I decided my lifestyle needed a serious reality check.

I came to the decision that it was time to swap the beer for trainers and the takeaways for healthy eating. I soon realised that healthy food and exercise will play an important role in building my future.

With focus and determination we all have the ability within us to make changes in our lives, and with a combination of exercise and healthy eating you can feel fit, have more energy and wind back the years.

Introduction 11

Although I am neither a chef nor personal trainer, I would like to share with you my journey and what I have learnt, and what has helped me to turn my life around.

So let's look at some of the most important areas to start with when you embark on your fitness and healthy eating journey.

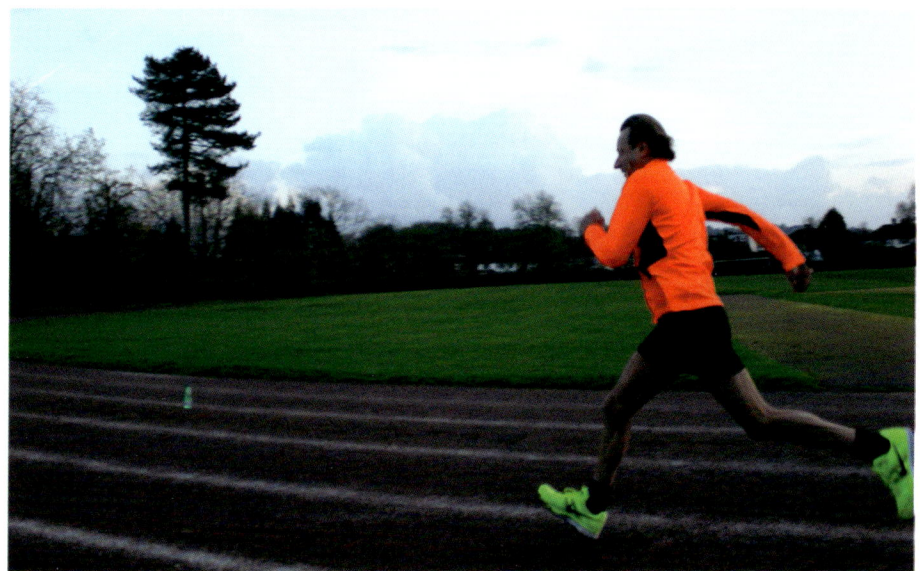

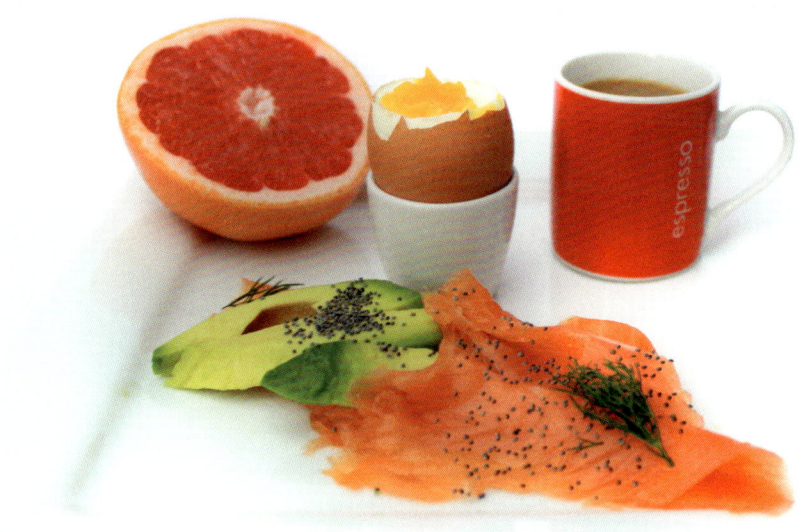

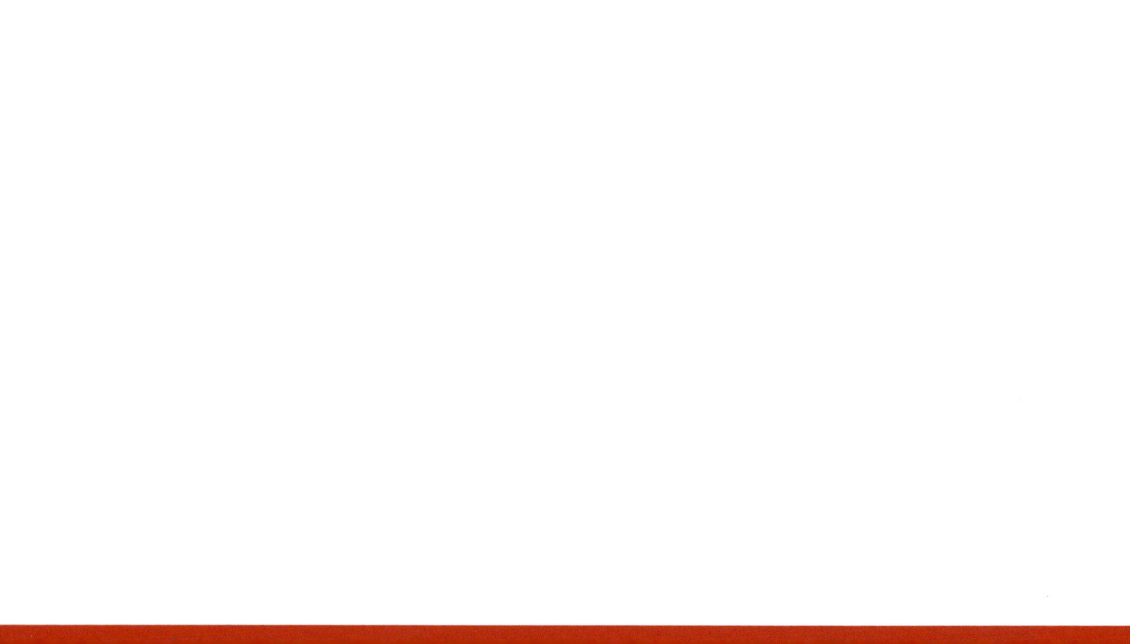

GET STARTED

1 ALCOHOL

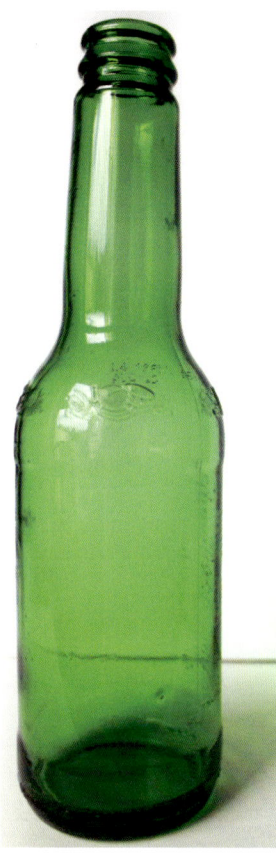

As men, we tend to find many reasons to drink and then drink way too much. It's very much a part of our culture as we grow up, and many of us have drunk to excess.

We see it as a great way to unwind and socialise, and for some of us it's part of our work to socialise with clients and colleagues alike. But while you can do this for a time in your younger years, it really doesn't take long for the effects of excess alcohol to start taking a toll on your body.

Alcohol is loaded with sugar which very quickly makes us fat, causing us to become out of shape and exhausted. Too much beer will give you the classic overhanging stomach, and it also moves its way around your back and gives you what is called back fat. You soon begin to look unattractive as you pile on the pounds, and the long-term effects can cause many illnesses such as diabetes, high blood pressure and liver disease.

Alcohol should be drunk in moderation, and you should aim to have at least three days a week without any, as this gives your body and liver time to flush out the harmful toxins.

TIPS FOR DRINKING

- Alternate alcoholic drinks with non-alcoholic drinks like water.
- Steer clear of premium beers which are loaded with sugar.
- A healthy meal or snack before you go out will line your stomach and slow the uptake of alcohol into your bloodstream.
- Swap the beer for red wine as this has antioxidants in it.
- Say no to shots.
- Say no to energy drinks.
- Say no to cocktails.
- If you drink spirits, then drink vodka with lemon or lime, as this has the fewest calories in it.

Alcohol in moderation is okay, but if you want to become a better, stronger and more focused person, the best advice I can give is to take a few days off; this, combined with healthy eating and exercise, will very quickly have you feeling much fitter in a small amount of time.

2 WATER

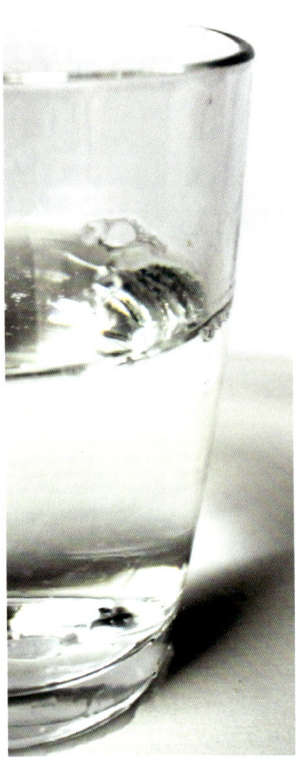

We should all aim to drink up to two litres of water a day, as this can:

- Increase energy and relieve fatigue
- Promote weight loss
- Flush out toxins
- Improve skin complexion
- Maintain regularity
- Boost your immune system
- Help relieve and prevent headaches and migraines
- Prevent cramp and sprains
- Improve your mood
- Promote a healthy heart

TIPS

- ✹ If you find it hard drinking water, start with drinking two glasses per day and every day increase by one glass.
- ✹ Before you go to bed, pimp your water by adding a lemon or lime and leaving it in the fridge overnight to infuse.

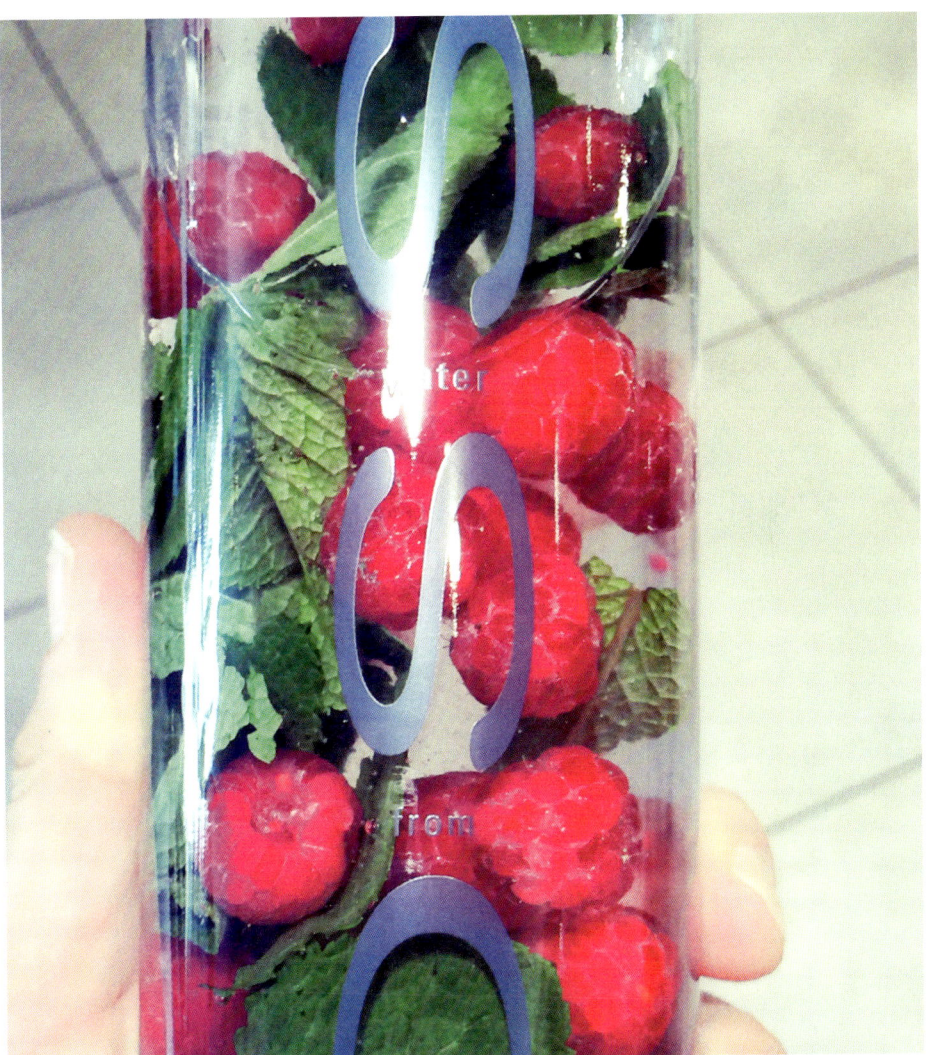

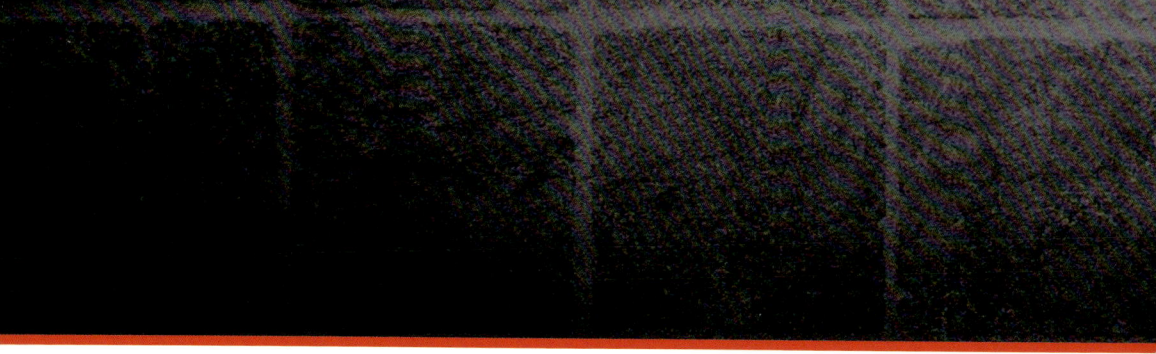

3 TOP FAT-BURNING FOODS

Certain foods have fat-burning elements and these help to fire up your natural metabolic rate, which means you burn off more calories at a faster rate. These are my top fat-burning foods for you to include in your weekly shopping:

- Salmon
- Quinoa
- Chillies
- Lentils
- Cinnamon
- Whole grains
- Brown rice
- Grapefruit
- Almonds
- Blueberries
- Eggs

3

4 PROCESSED FOODS

Today's supermarkets are full of processed foods. Don't be fooled by the way products are displayed and don't let yourself be tricked into thinking products are low in fat, ocean fresh, high in fibre, etc., when they really aren't. The clever use of pictures can make you believe you are buying healthy products. Many times the food has come a long way from its natural environment and has been stripped of its natural vitamins and augmented with artificial colouring, extra sugar and salt to preserve its shelf life.

WHAT TO AVOID

- White bread
- Sugar
- Ready meals
- Dried pasta
- White rice
- Breakfast cereals
- Tinned food
- Cakes
- Biscuits
- Crisps
- Sweets
- Fruit juices

Processed Foods

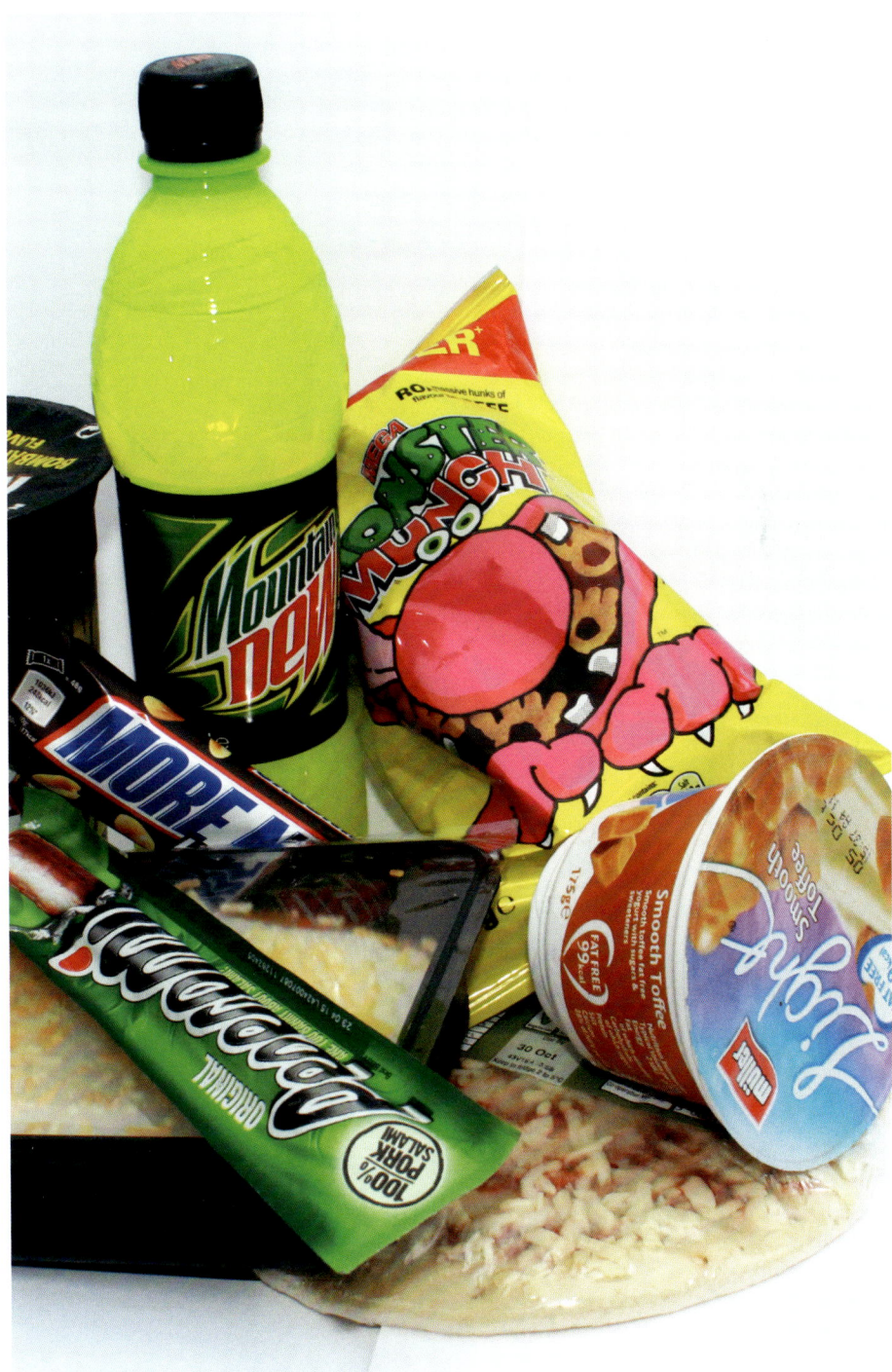

5 SUGAR

Health experts are now saying sugar is as dangerous as alcohol and smoking, and that this is the leading cause of obesity, diabetes and many other serious health conditions. Sugar is hidden in most food and drinks, even the ones that supermarkets display as low in fat or healthy.

Health experts also say that 40% of the sugar you eat turns into fat. Cut back, and you will start to feel slimmer and have more energy which will prevent those sugar slumps.

HIDDEN SUGAR BOMBS

- Breakfast cereal bars
- Fruit juice
- Alcohol
- White carbs
- White refined sugar
- Low-fat foods
- Fizzy drinks
- Pasta sauces
- Fruit yoghurt
- Agave
- Sweets
- Energy drinks

Sugar

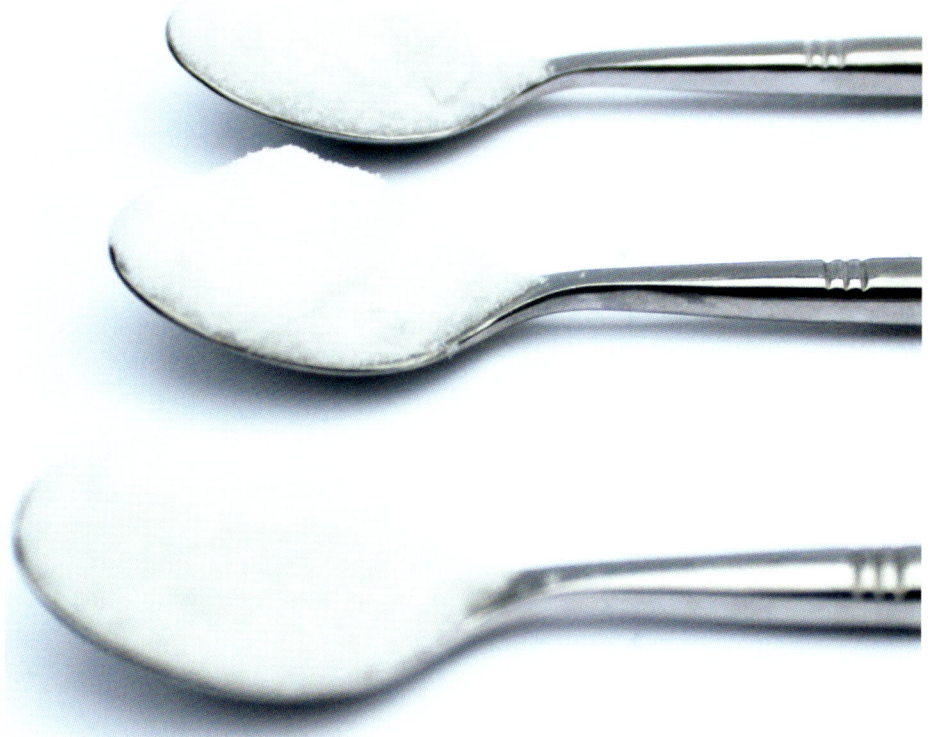

6 NUTRITION

THE FARM SHOP

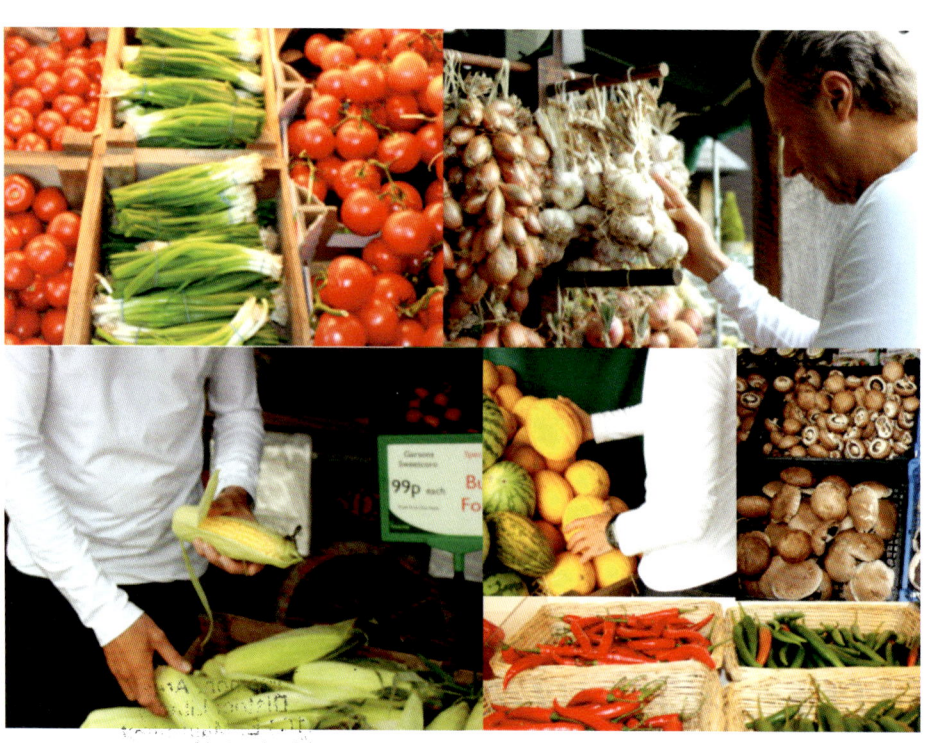

If you are fortunate enough to live near a farm shop, I highly recommend you shop there. Farmers' shops are organic and will be full of the nutrition you need. They have an amazing variety of fresh fruit and vegetables and, quite simply, their food tastes so much better and is so much better for you.

TIPS

- If you use your local supermarket, try to only buy fresh and unprocessed food.
- Buy your meat from a local butcher, as this will be fresher and not full of toxins.
- Only buy fruit and vegetables that are in season.

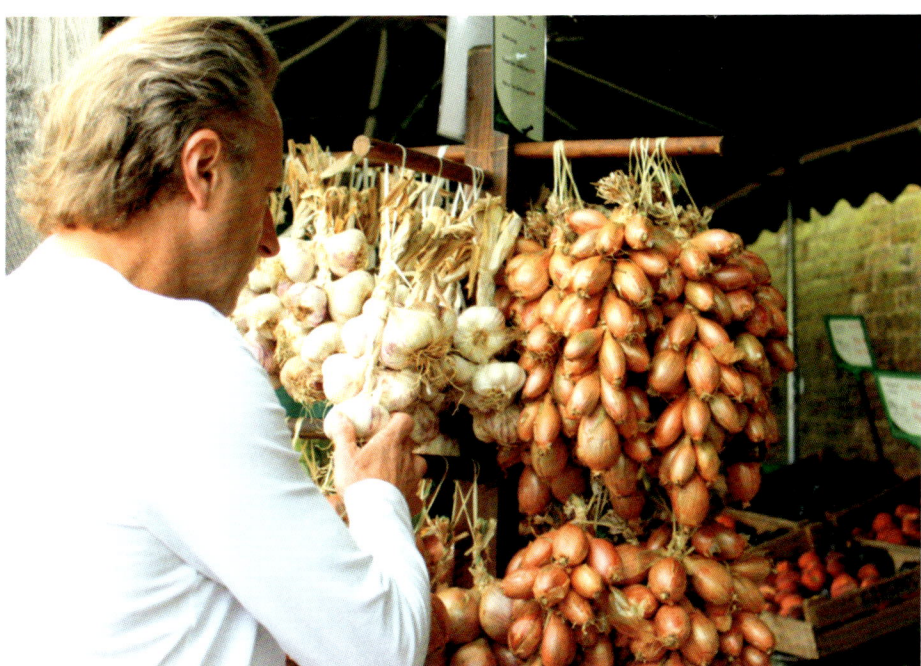

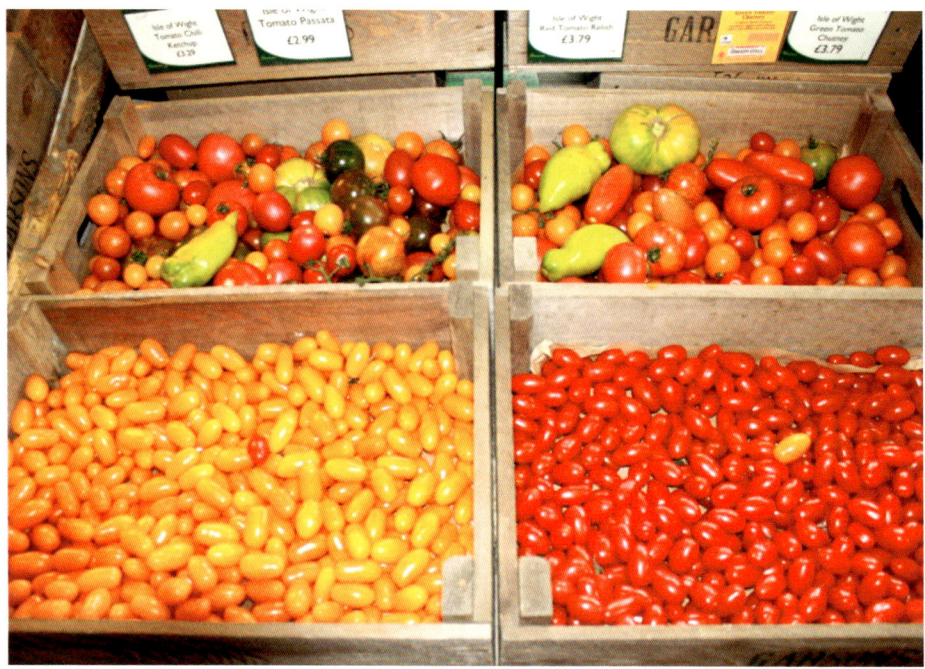

PROTEIN

Protein is an essential part of your diet as it is responsible for repairing and building your muscles as well as keeping your immune system fighting fit.

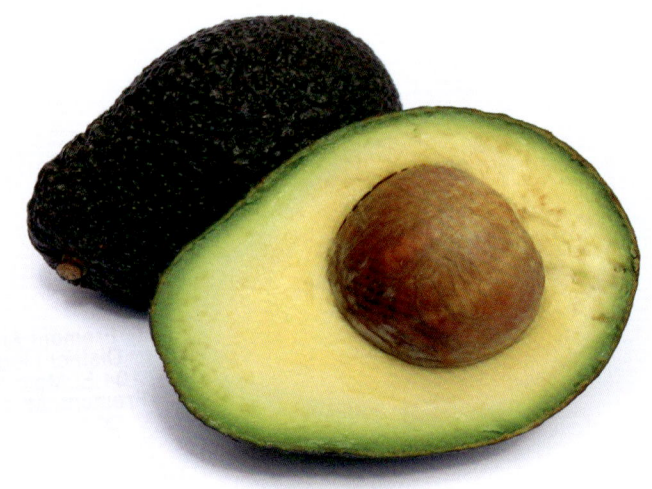

YOUR SHOPPING LIST SHOULD INCLUDE SOME OF THE FOLLOWING:

- Nuts
- Fish
- Eggs
- Beef
- Turkey
- Avocado
- Chicken

TIP

- Try to include a small amount of protein with every meal, as this will keep you fuller for longer and help build muscle.

CARBOHYDRATES

Carbs are a good source of energy as long as we eat the right carbs. Good carbs are those that have not lost their nutrients, unlike bad carbs which have been stripped of nutrients for a longer shelf life in your local supermarket.

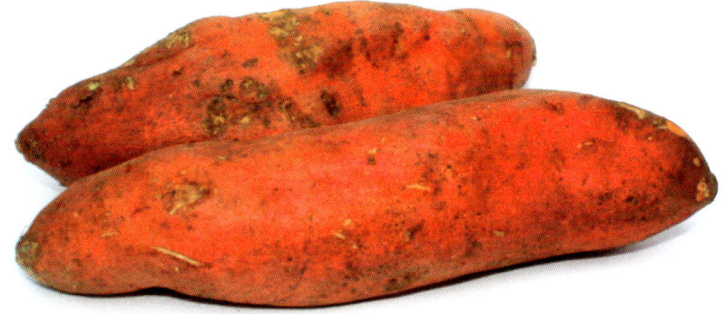

- Sweet potato
- Brown rice
- Quinoa
- Chickpeas
- Peas
- Oats
- Berries
- Chia seeds
- Zucchini
- Whole-grain pasta

TIP

An example of turning good carbs into bad carbs is brown rice being stripped of its fibre and turned white, and having sugar and chemicals added. It may have a longer shelf life, but now it is stripped of all of its goodness.

Fats

Fats are an important part of a healthy diet as long as we stick to natural fats, and not man-made fats. Fats help you absorb vitamins such as A, E, D and K.

HEALTHY FATS CAN BE FOUND IN THE FOLLOWING:

- Salmon
- Avocado
- Extra virgin olive oil
- Nuts and seeds
- Eggs
- Tuna
- Sardines
- Mackerel
- Trout

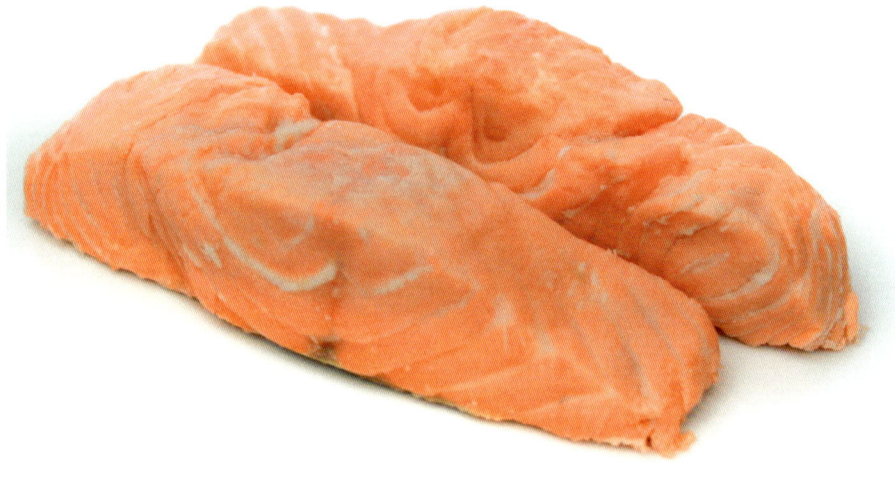

FIBRE

Fibre plays an important role in our daily diet; it helps the digestive system process food and absorbs nutrients. It is filling and keeps us fuller for longer, helping us to maintain a healthy weight.

- Sweet corn
- Kidney beans
- Chickpeas
- Avocado
- Lentils
- Pears
- Oatmeal
- Raspberries

VEGETABLES

These are the biggest sources of natural vitamins and minerals you can find; you should try to include at least three portions of these in your daily diet:

- Asparagus
- Spinach
- Kale
- Green beans
- Peas
- Broccoli
- Zucchini
- Leeks
- Carrots
- Peppers
- Radish
- Brussels sprouts
- Sweet potato

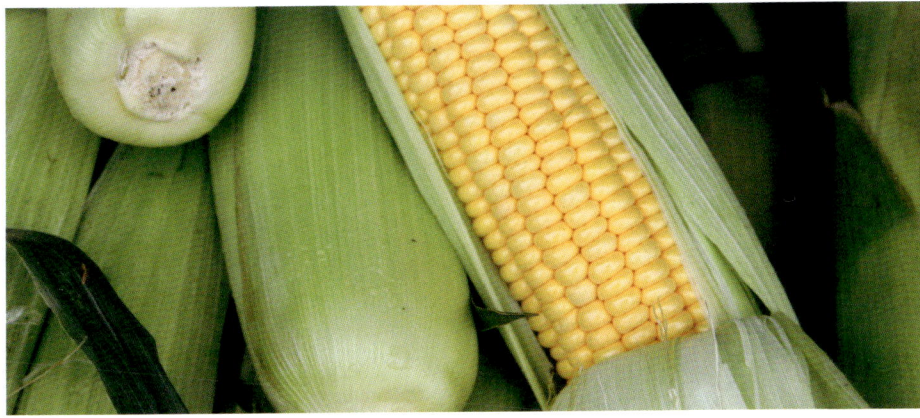

FRUITS

Fruits contain vitamins and minerals and are high in antioxidants. Even though some fruits are high in sugar, it is all-natural sugar. Aim to have two pieces of fruit a day.

- Strawberries
- Blueberries
- Raspberries
- Bananas
- Apples
- Melon
- Grapefruit
- Kiwi
- Oranges
- Pineapples
- Passion fruit
- Plums
- Peaches
- Nectarines
- Cherries
- Avocado

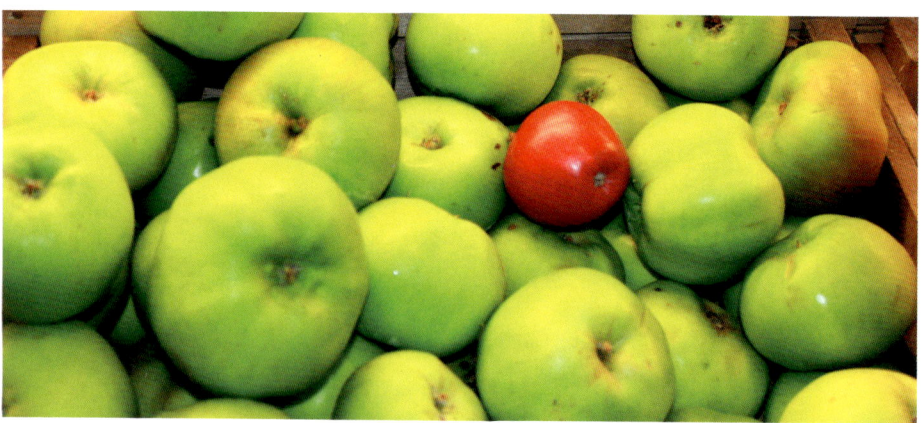

NUTS AND SEEDS

Nuts and seeds have a myriad of health benefits and also make a great, quick snack. They are an excellent source of fibre and vitamins, which help keep your body running like a well-oiled machine.

- Hazelnuts
- Almonds
- Pistachio nuts
- Cashews
- Walnuts
- Pecans
- Brazil nuts
- Sunflower seeds
- Pumpkin seeds
- Chia seeds
- Flax seeds
- Linseeds

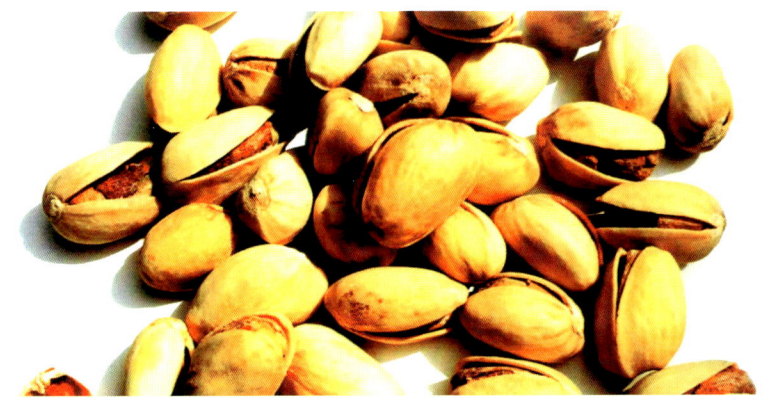

HERBS

It is important to use fresh herbs in all of your foods where possible. They enhance the taste and can turn a simple meal into a mouth-watering dish. Herbs are not only just flavour boosters; they carry many health benefits which help our bodies to fight against germs and toxins and to boost immunity levels.

- Basil
- Mint
- Coriander
- Sage
- Chives
- Dill
- Parsley
- Tarragon
- Thyme
- Oregano
- Lemon grass
- Rosemary
- Turmeric

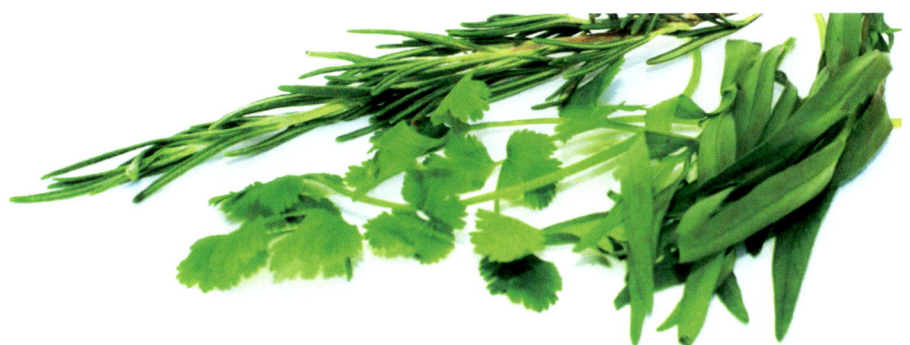

Now you have a list of some of the food you should include in your weekly shopping, so it's time to get cooking!

RECIPES

7 BREAKFAST

We have all heard it before, but breakfast really is the most important meal of the day. It can help control your weight and boost your energy levels throughout the day. It can improve your mood and keep you from craving more processed foods within a couple of hours.

Clever marketing has fooled us into accepting that conventional breakfasts such as toast and marmalade, cereal and fruit juice are nutritious, healthy and a great way to start your day.

Sadly these have no health benefits at all, as they are over processed and loaded with sugar, resulting in fat stored on your waistline.

So what is a healthy breakfast? A healthy breakfast should be easy to create, with some imagination and careful planning. You could have a simple egg breakfast with some nuts and fruit or you could have a super protein smoothie. If it's cereal you like, then create your own by taking a trip to the local health store and buying your own ingredients.

By making the right choices in your breakfast, you will lift your energy levels and also help burn fat.

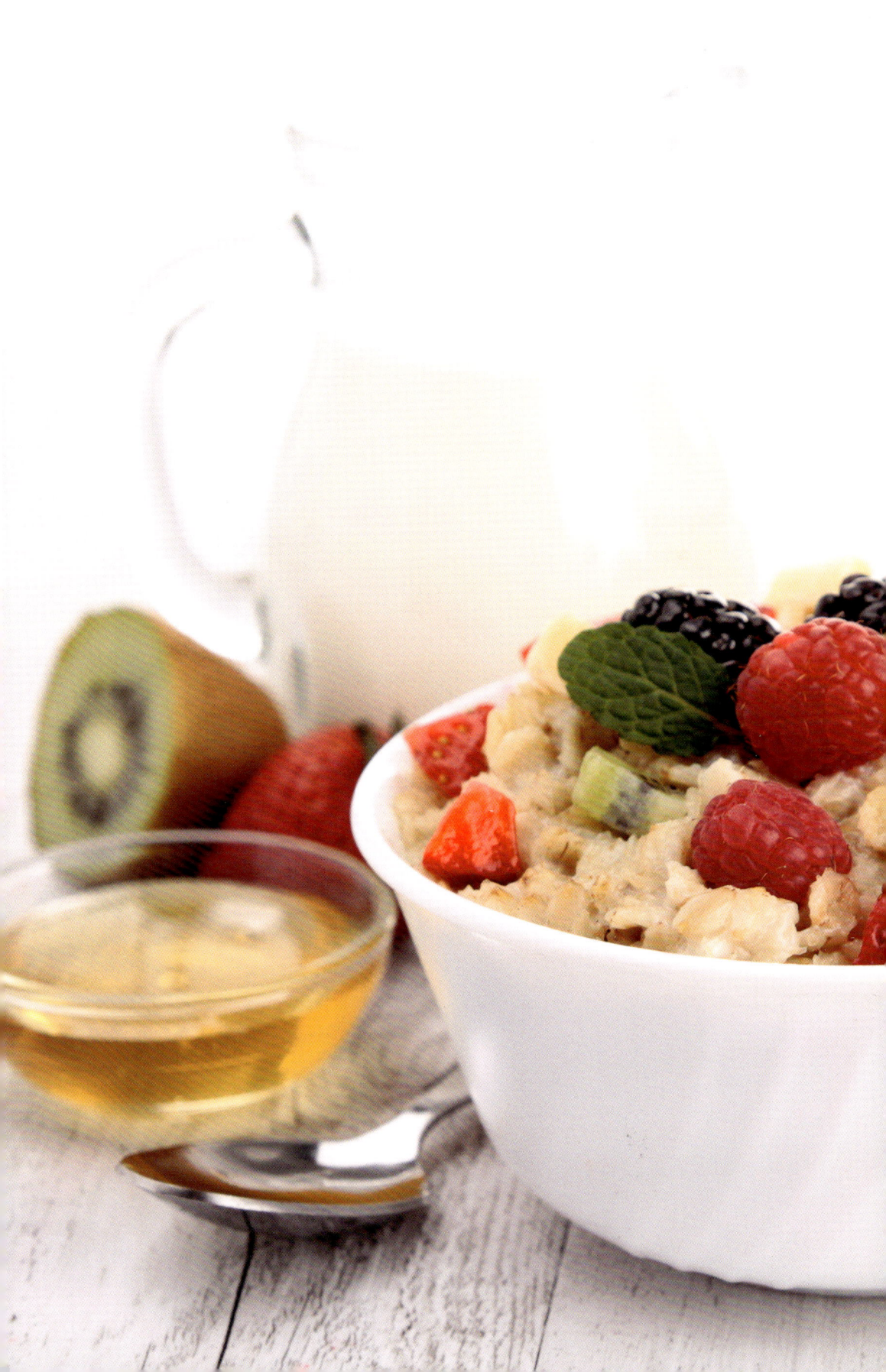

TIP

✺ Taking some time to dress and present your breakfast will make it look and taste better, and it's a great way to impress yourself.

ENERGY-BOOSTING BREAKFAST

INGREDIENTS

A handful of oats

A good dollop of natural yoghurt

A spoonful of chia seeds

Kiwi

Blackberries

Blueberries

Strawberry

INSTRUCTIONS

Start with a small layer of oats, add a few dollops of natural yoghurt and a spoonful of chia seeds, and dress with the remaining fruit.

Simple to make, and packs in all the nutrients you need to start your day!

TIP

CHIA SEEDS CONTAIN 7 TIMES MORE VITAMIN C THAN AN ORANGE.

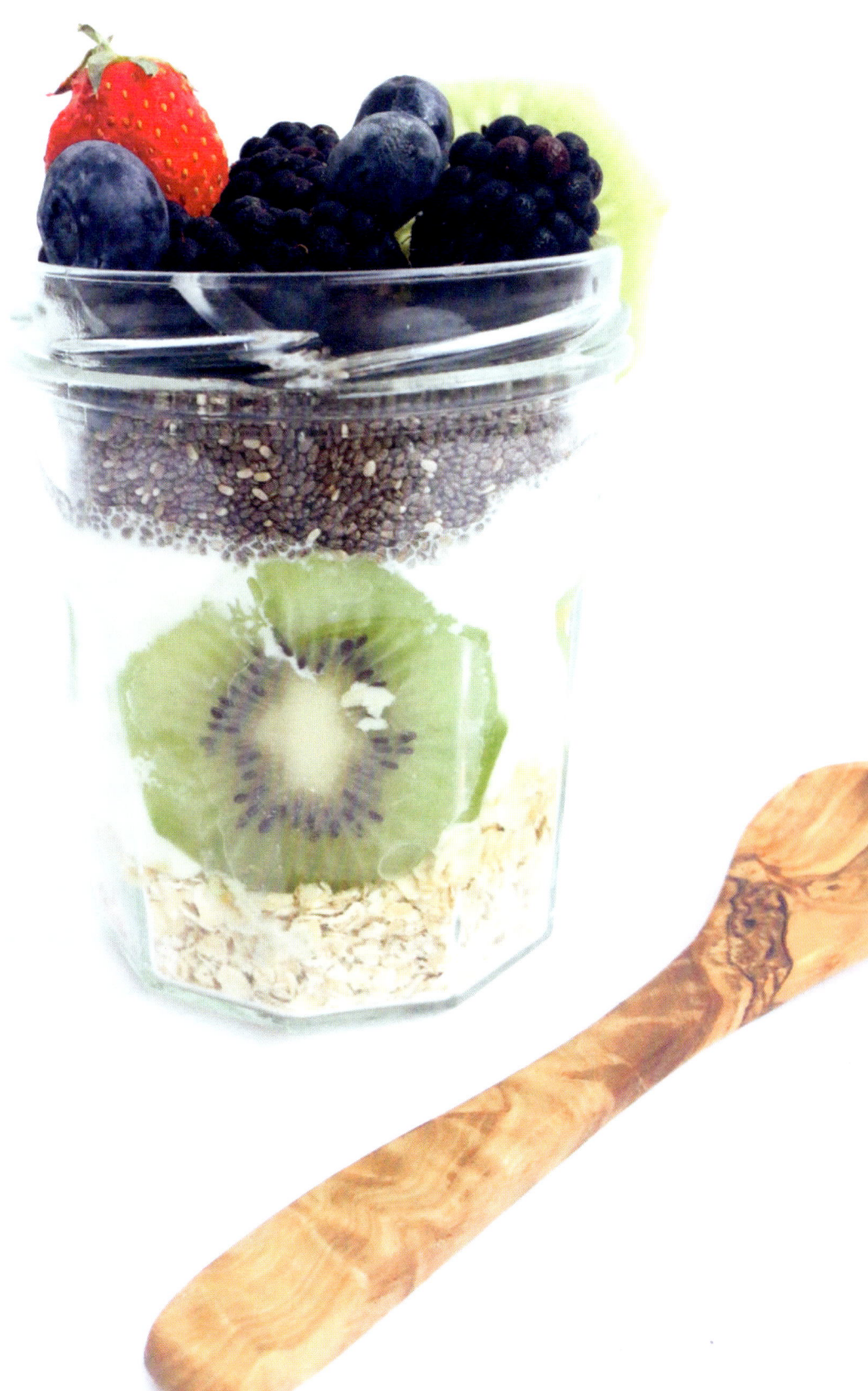

Men´s Fit **Kitchen**

HONEY, NUTS AND YOGHURT

INGREDIENTS

Natural yoghurt

A few slices of banana

A handful of raspberries

Mixed nuts

Honey

INSTRUCTIONS

Take a good helping of yoghurt and mix in the rest of the ingredients.

TIP

YOU CAN DRIZZLE VANILLA ESSENCE OR SPRINKLE CINNAMON OVER THIS FOR EXTRA TASTE.

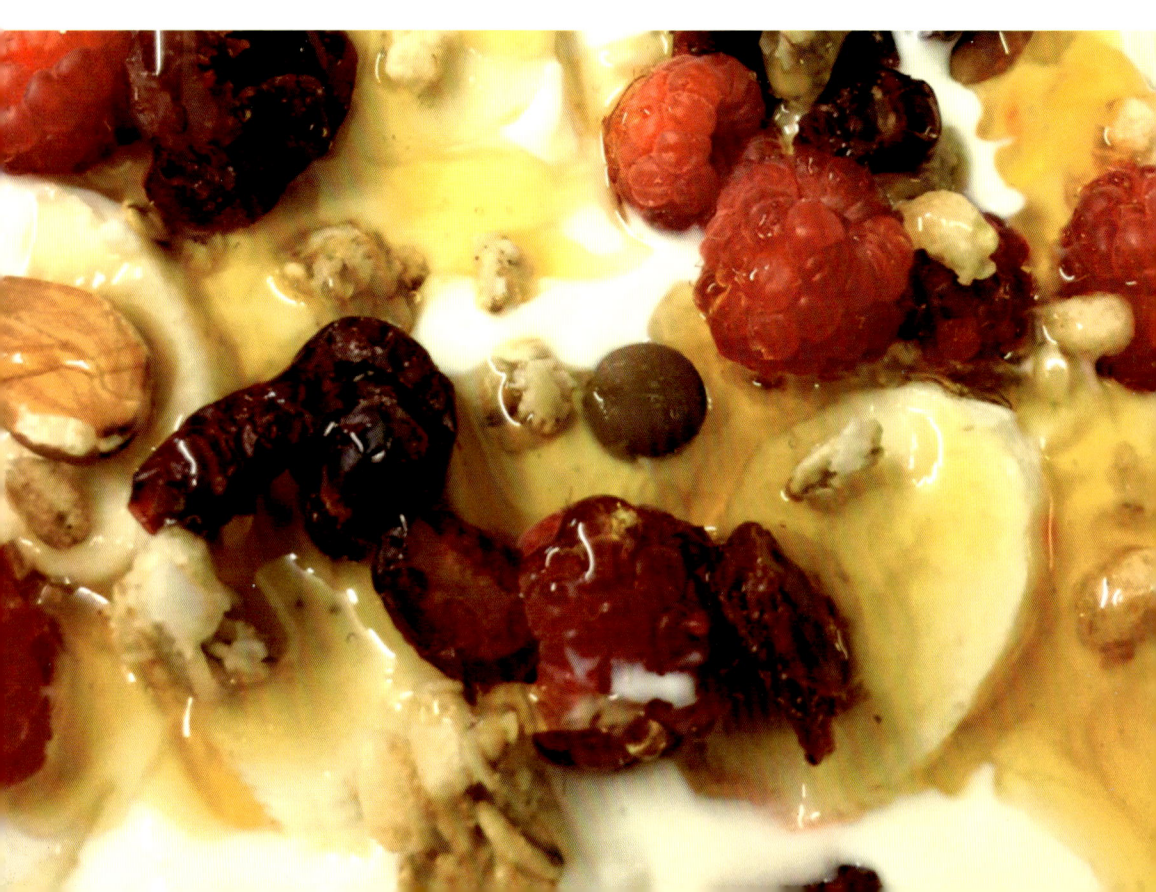

POWER PORRIDGE

INGREDIENTS

Oats

Raspberries

Banana

Chia seeds

Milk or yoghurt

INSTRUCTIONS

Start with a good layer of oats, dress with the raspberries, banana and chia seeds, and mix with any kind of milk or natural yoghurt.

TIP

BE CREATIVE AND TAKE THE TIME TO DRESS YOUR FOOD LIKE YOU ARE STARRING IN MASTER CHEF.

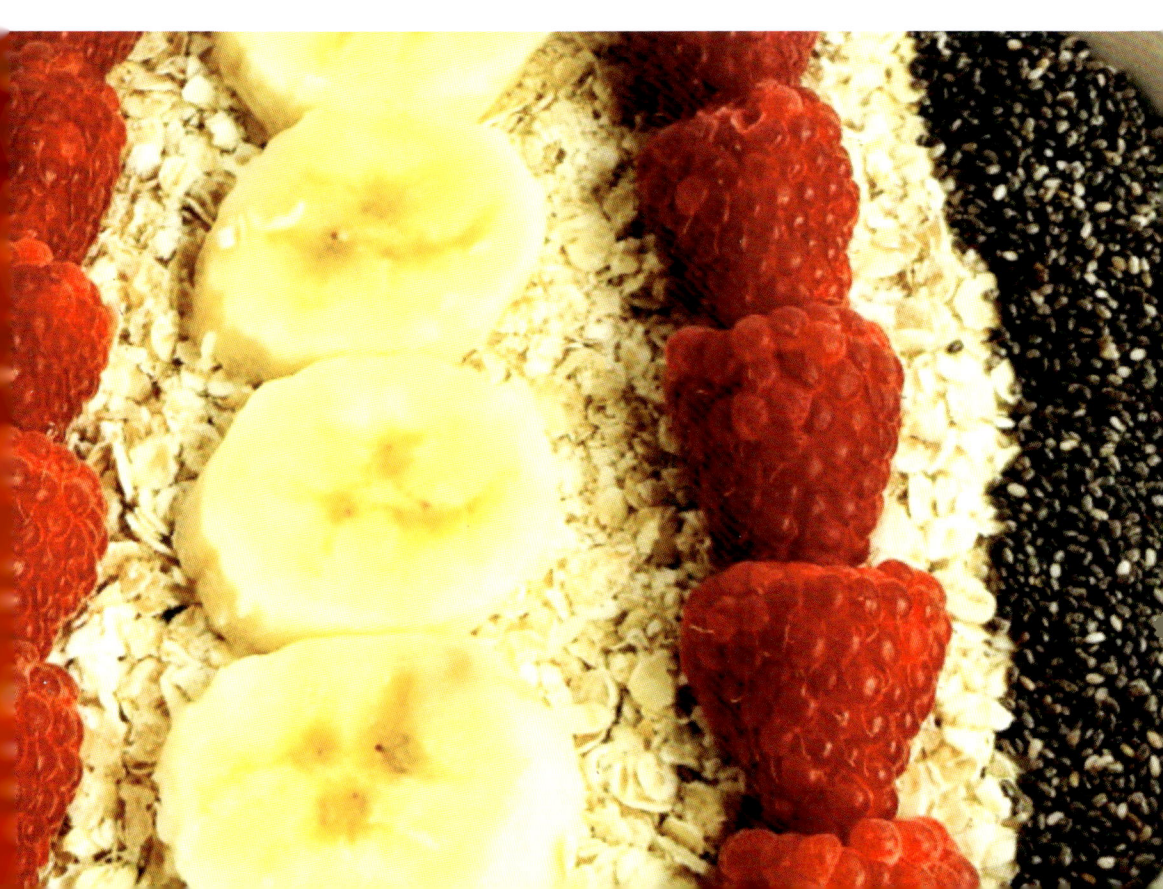

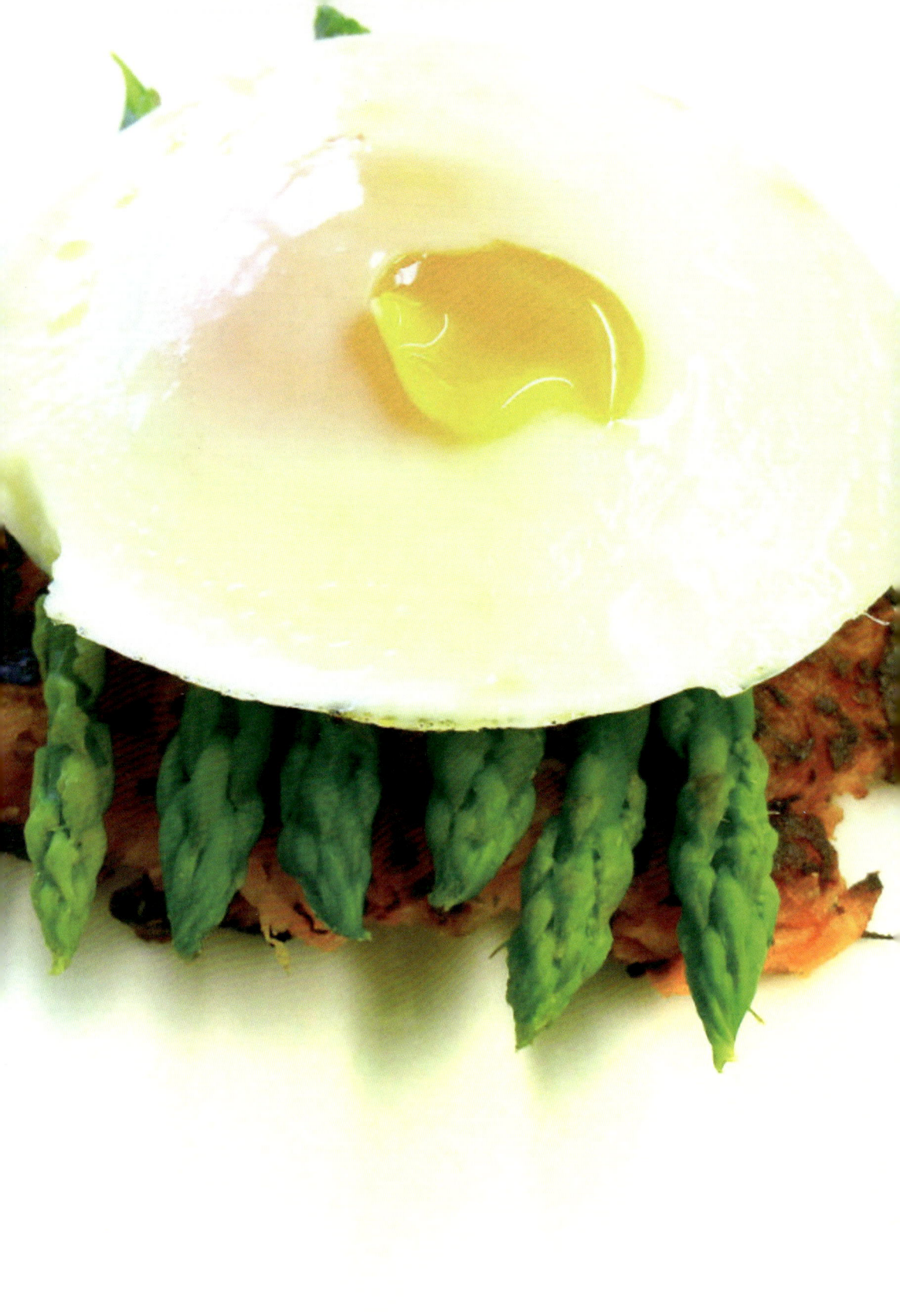

SWEET POTATO HASH

INGREDIENTS

1 egg

6 asparagus stalks

1 small sweet potato, peeled

Coriander

Olive oil

INSTRUCTIONS

Parboil the sweet potato for 5 minutes. Drain and mash roughly. Add a good handful of coriander and season to taste.

Once the mash is cool enough to handle, form it into a thin patty. Transfer to a frying pan with a small drizzle of olive oil, and cook on a low heat for 3 minutes on each side.

Meanwhile bring a pot of water to a boil. Drop the asparagus in, and simmer for about 3-4 minutes.

In a small frying pan add a drizzle of olive oil, crack an egg, and fry for 3-4 minutes.

Carefully stack all components on a plate and enjoy.

OPEN-FACED BREAKFAST CLUB SANDWICH

INGREDIENTS

1 slice of wholemeal toast

A handful of rocket leaves

Half of an avocado, sliced

1 egg

1 medium tomato, sliced

A good slice of smoked salmon

Salt and pepper to taste

INSTRUCTIONS

Bring a pot of water to a boil, add egg, and simmer for about 4 minutes.

Toast the bread, and dress with rocket, salmon, tomato and avocado. Peel the boiled egg, then place on top and season.

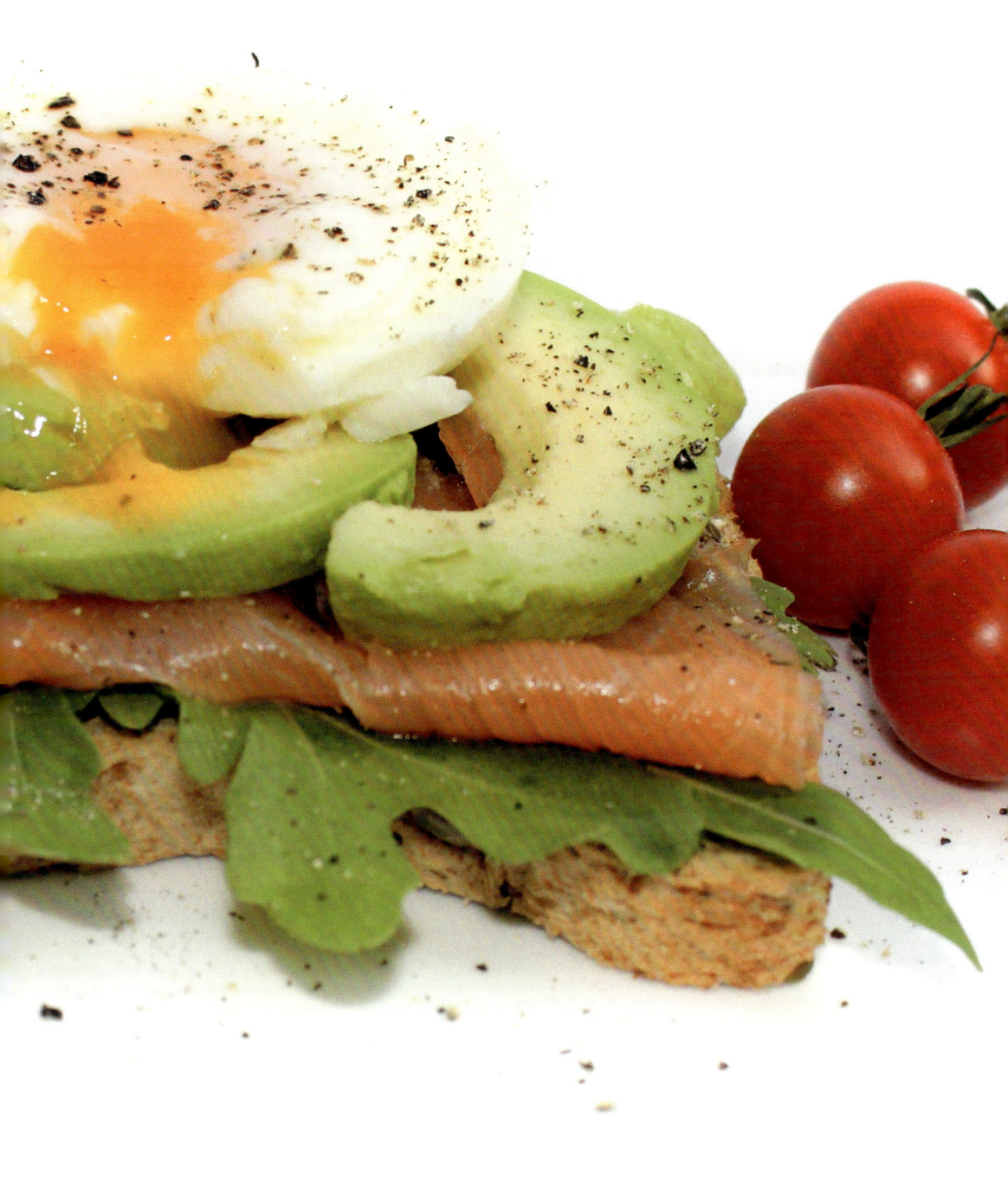

EGGS

Eggs can be boiled, poached, fried or scrambled, but however they're prepared, eggs fulfil a significant function in your breakfast. They are packed with protein and nutrient rich, which can help you get fit and healthy. Eggs can play an important role in making a super healthy protein-packed breakfast.

Your only limitation when it comes to cooking eggs is going to be your imagination!

- Plain boiled eggs can make a great breakfast or a perfect addition to your lunchtime salad.
- Try adding salmon, ham or spinach to scrambled eggs.
- Get creative and make an omelette. There are no rules here, just a little imagination, like adding onion, peppers, mushrooms, and a little cheese.
- Poached eggs are perfect on their own or with a slice of wholemeal toast and a small portion of white fish and asparagus.

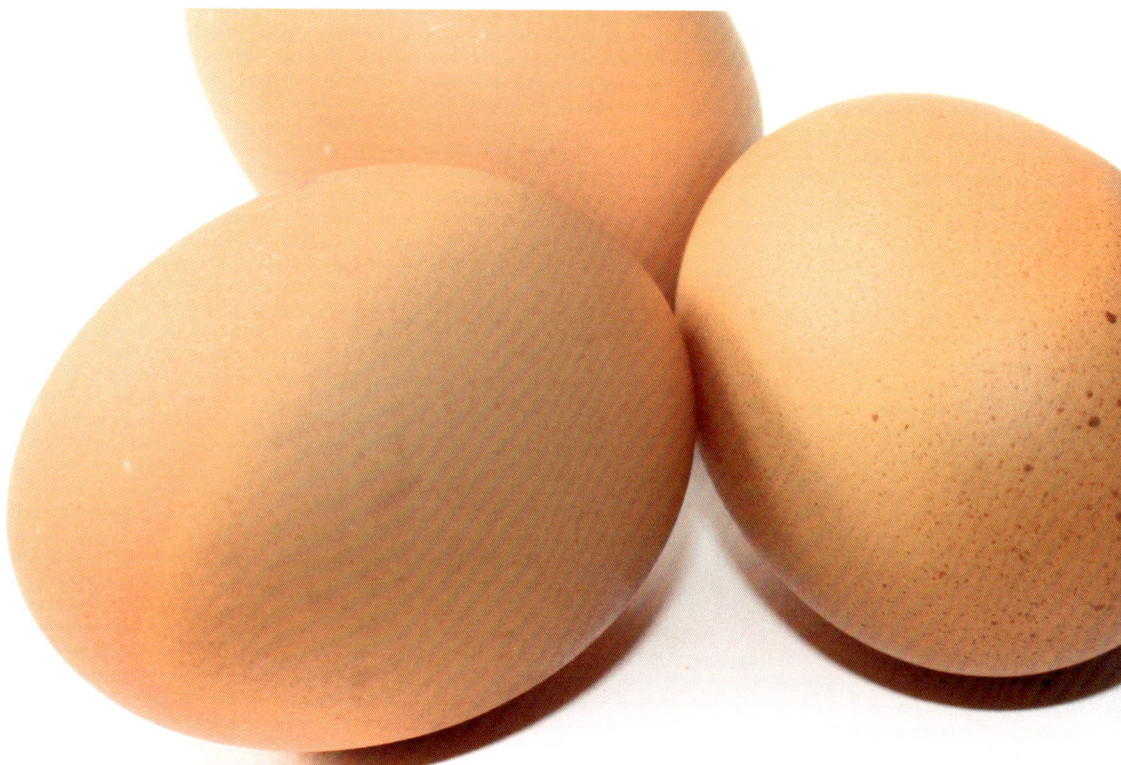

A ROUGH GUIDE TO COOKING EGGS

BOILED EGGS

Bring a pot of water to a boil and add egg. Cook to desired consistency using the following guide:

1. Soft middle: 4 minutes
2. Semi-soft: 7 minutes
3. Hard-boiled: 8 minutes

POACHED EGGS

Bring a pot of water to a boil, add a small splash of vinegar, and then lower the heat to a gentle simmer. Crack an egg into a cup and gently pour into the pan. Simmer for just over 4 minutes.

SCRAMBLED EGGS

Crack 2 eggs into a small bowl. Add two tablespoons of milk and freshly ground black pepper. Whisk the mixture with a fork.

Melt a small knob of butter in a frying pan. Add the egg mixture and gently stir until cooked.

Men´s Fit **Kitchen**

POWER PROTEIN OMELETTE

INGREDIENTS

2 eggs

2 tbsp. milk

Salt and pepper to taste

1 small knob of butter

Half of an avocado

1 slice of Smoked salmon

1 small red onion, diced

1 tomato, diced

A small portion of Feta cheese, crumbled

INSTRUCTIONS

Crack the eggs into a bowl, add a small dash of milk, mix and season.

Melt butter in a frying pan, and pour the mixture in.

Cook for two minutes on each side, and then slide onto a plate.

Carefully add the rest of the ingredients, fold in half and enjoy.

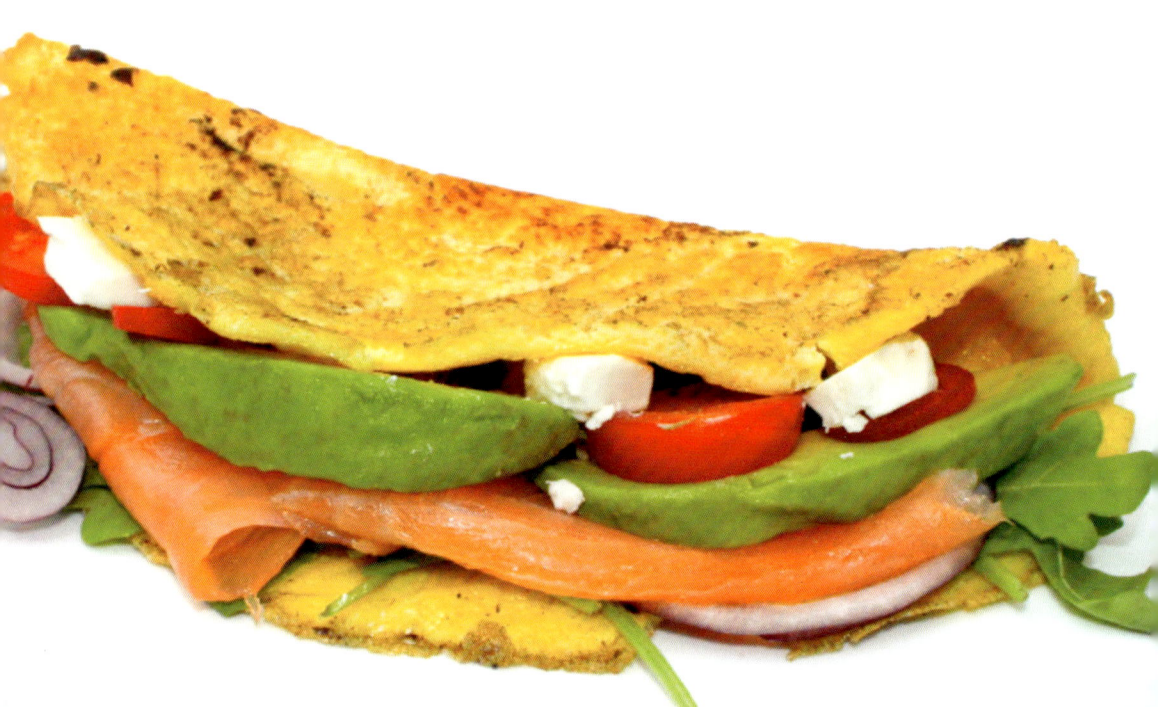

EGG AND ASPARAGUS

INGREDIENTS

1 boiled egg

5 asparagus spears

INSTRUCTIONS

Bring a pot of water to a boil. Place asparagus in boiling water and cook for 3 minutes. Drain and place on plate

Place the boiled egg in an egg cup, slice the top off and breakfast is served.

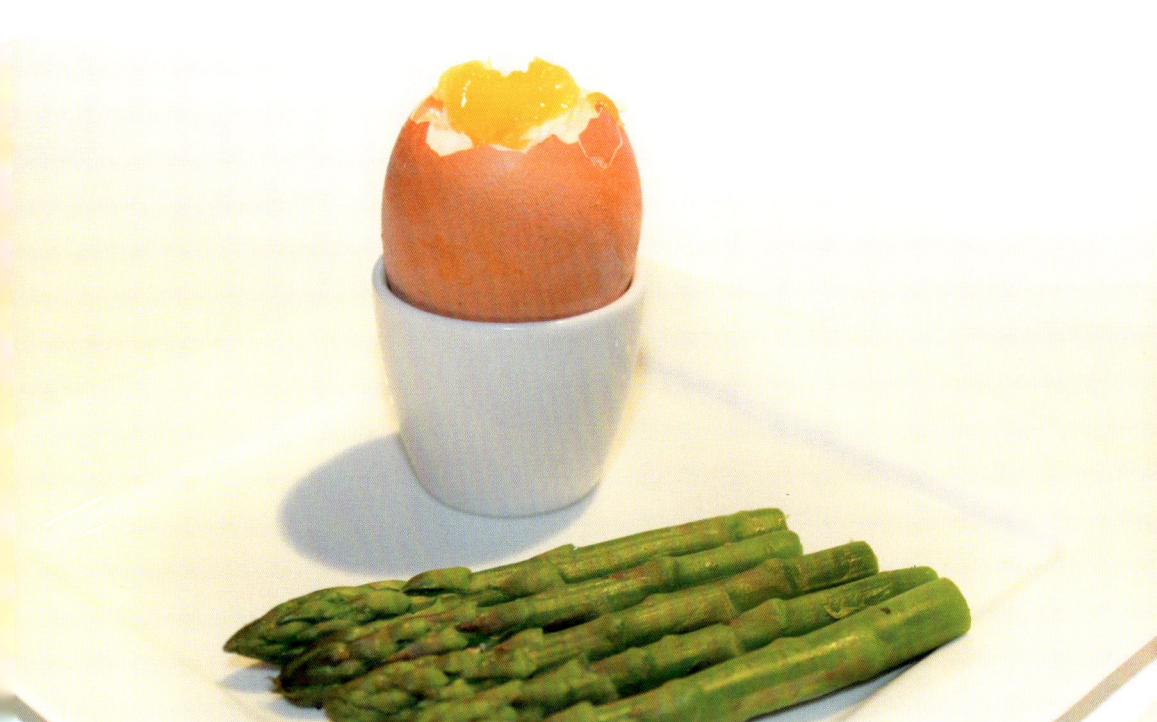

ALMOND PORRIDGE

INGREDIENTS

1 cup of oats

2 cups of Almond milk

1 kiwi

6 raspberrys

Honey (optional)

INSTRUCTIONS

Place oats in a saucepan and pour in the milk. Bring to a boil, lower temperature and simmer for 4-5 minutes, stirring from time to time to make sure it doesn't stick to the bottom of the pan.

Pour oatmeal into a bowl and dress with kiwi and raspberry. If desired, drizzle with honey.

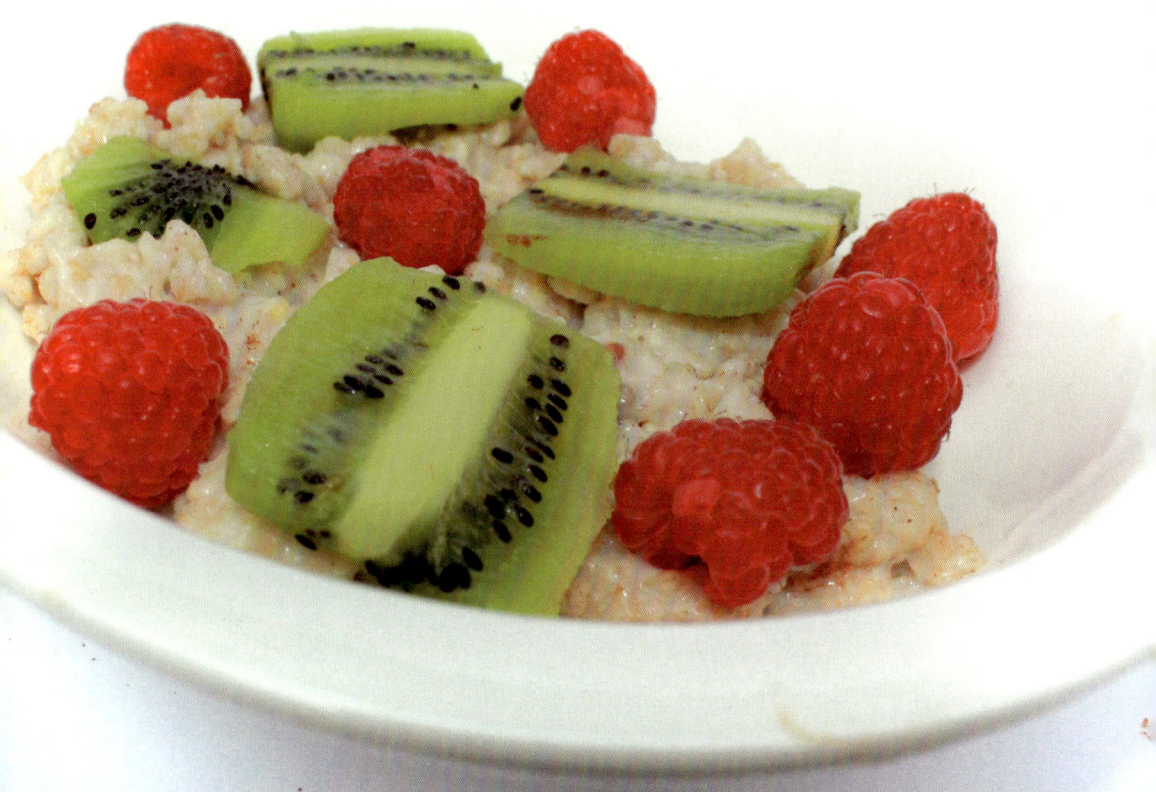

OPEN-FACED PEANUT BUTTER CRUNCH

INGREDIENTS

1 slice of wholemeal bread, toasted

Peanut butter

1 small banana, sliced

Hazelnuts, crushed

INSTRUCTIONS

Spread toasted bread with a good helping of peanut butter and top with sliced banana. Dress with crushed hazelnuts.

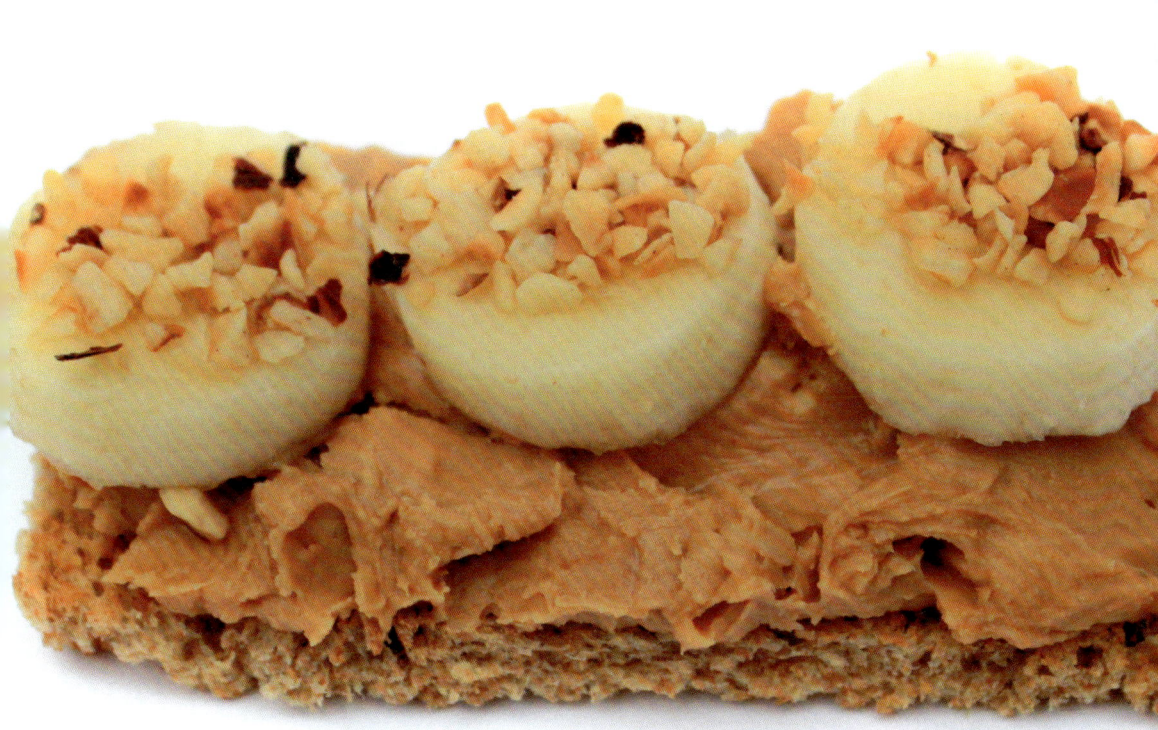

PROTEIN PUNCH

INGREDIENTS

2 small sardines

1 slice of wholemeal bread, toasted

Splash of lemon juice

Black pepper to taste

INSTRUCTIONS

Top the toasted bread with sardines and a drop of lemon juice. Season with black pepper to taste.

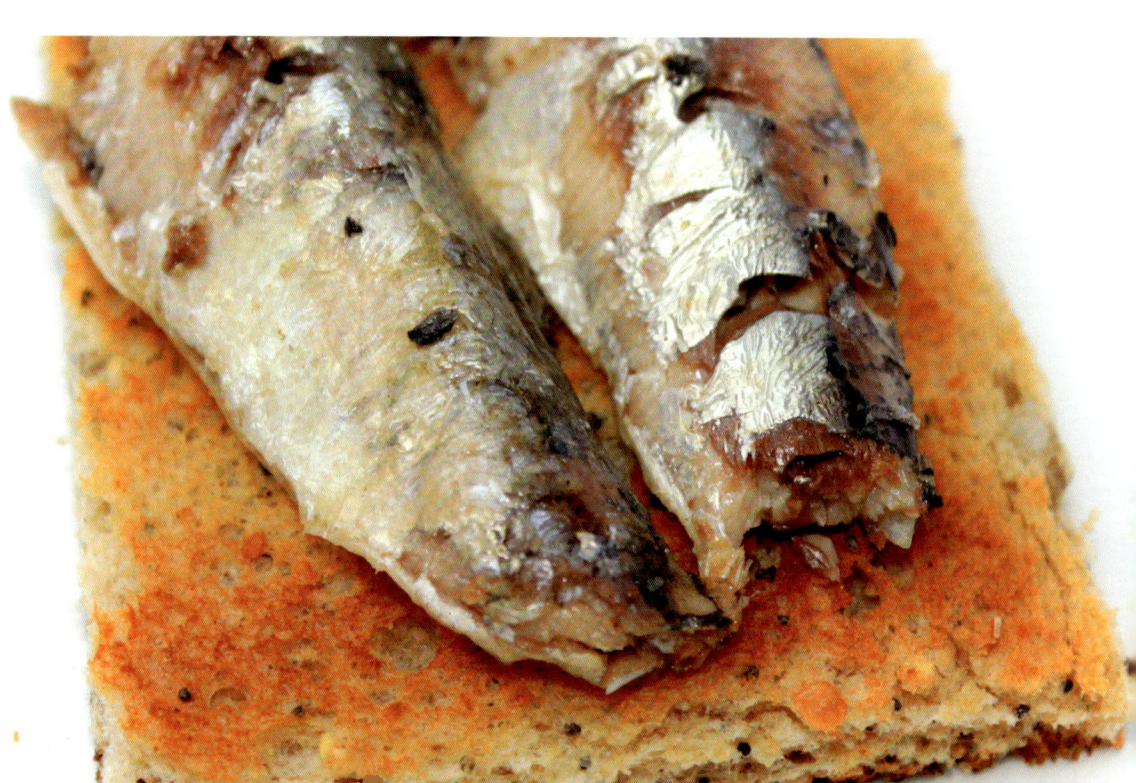

BANANA PANCAKES

INGREDIENTS

1 egg

1 small, very ripe banana, mashed

Coconut oil

Kiwi

Greek yoghurt

Pomegranate seeds

INSTRUCTIONS

Stir together the egg and the mashed banana.

Heat a frying pan with a small amount of coconut oil. Add half of the mixture to the pan and slowly cook, keeping it together in a nice circle. Cook for 2 minutes and flip to the other side for a further 2 minutes. Remove from the pan and set aside.

Add the rest of the mixture and repeat.

Place both pancakes on a plate and dress with a good helping of Greek yoghurt, a few slices of kiwi and a few pomegranate seeds

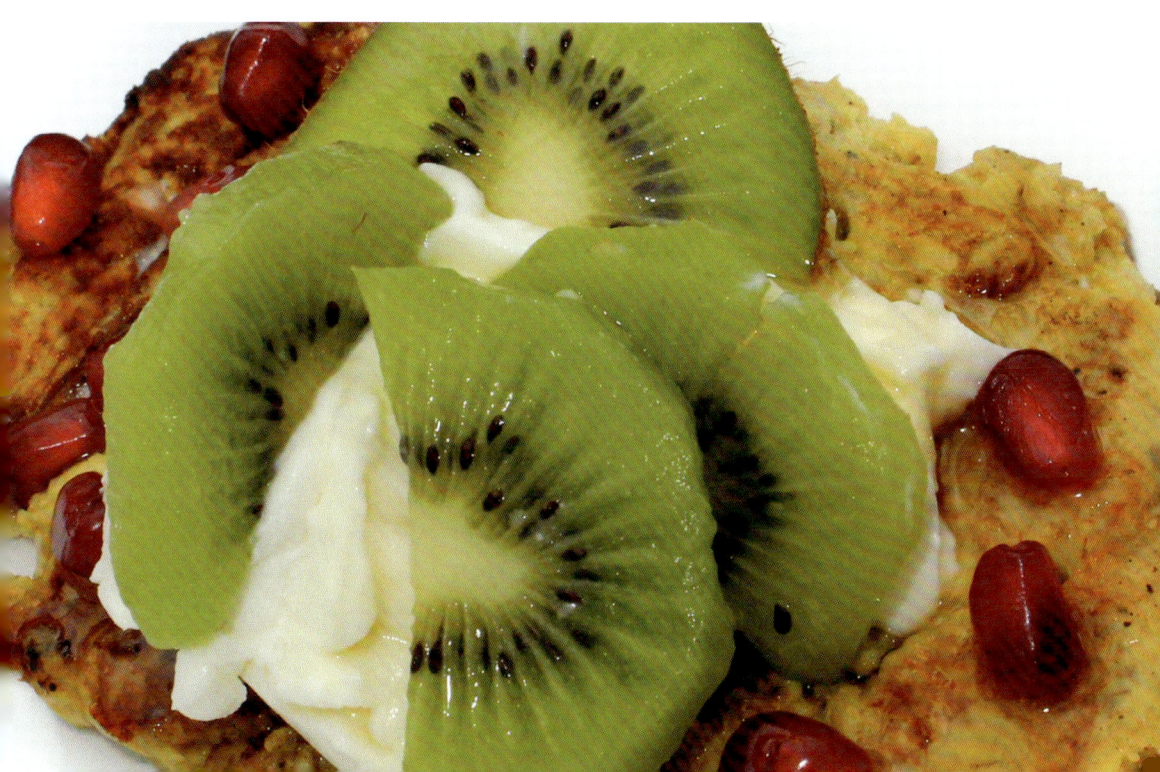

SALMON-WRAPPED ASPARAGUS

INGREDIENTS

6 asparagus spears

6 small slices of smoked salmon

Splash of lemon juice

Black pepper to taste

INSTRUCTIONS

Bring a pot of water to a boil. Add the asparagus and cook for 3 minutes. Drain and allow the asparagus to cool slightly.

Carefully wrap the smoked salmon around the asparagus, drizzle with a squeeze of lemon and season with black pepper to taste.

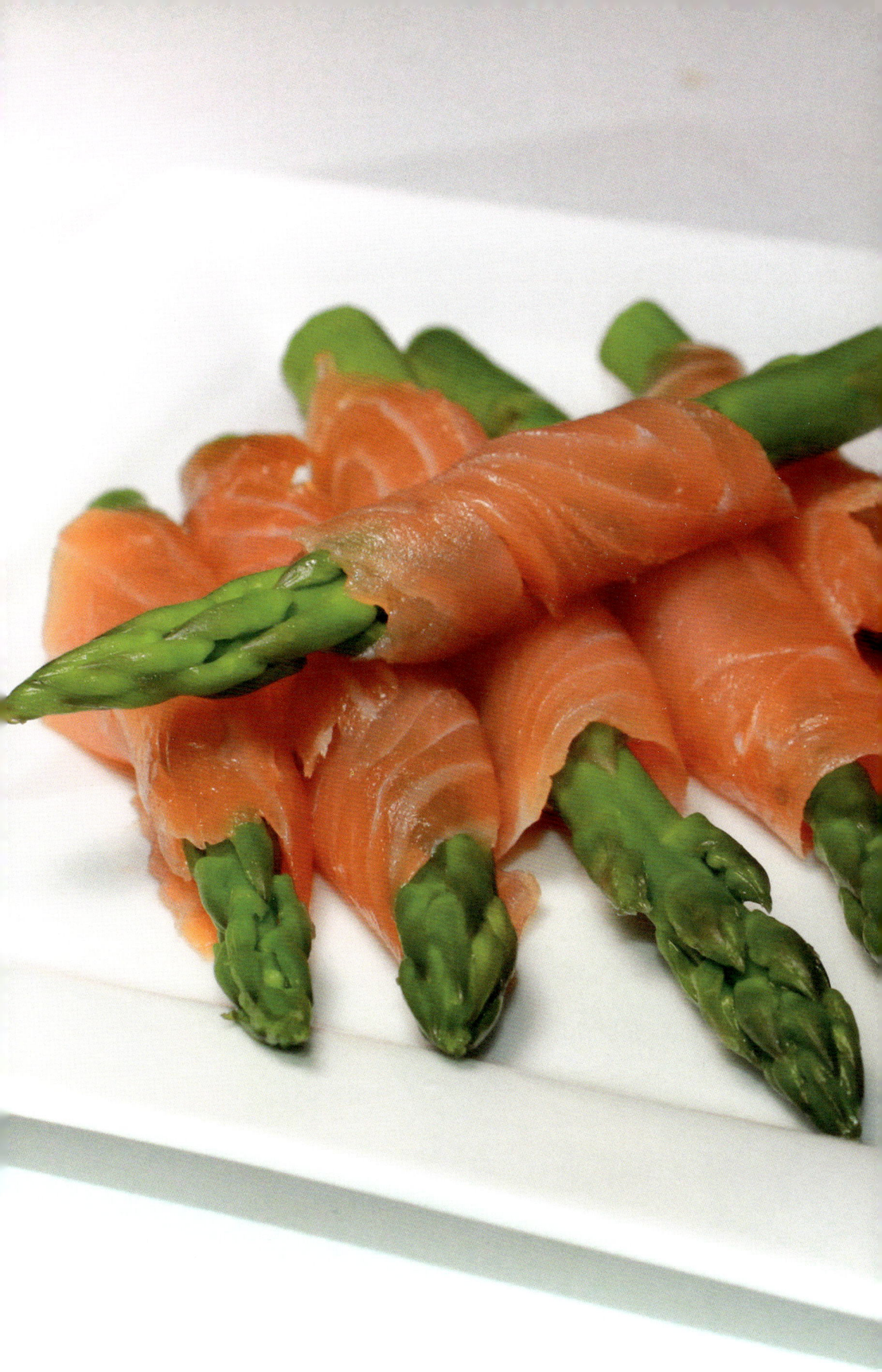

8 LUNCH

Eating a healthy lunch is important for many reasons. Food gives us energy. A nutrient-packed lunch will help you avoid that mid-afternoon crash.

Avoiding lunch will leave you hungry and likely to search for a quick fix in the form of chocolate, crisps and cakes which have little nutritional value and are full of sugar—one of the greatest ways to pile on the pounds.

FOODS TO AVOID

- Pre-packaged sandwiches
- Ready meals
- Crisps
- Cakes

FOODS TO INCLUDE

- Protein: chicken, fish, eggs
- Good fat: avocado, nuts and seeds
- Vegetables: any green leaves, peppers, cucumber, broccoli, tomatoes, and radishes

Lunch does not have to be boring; with a little imagination and careful planning, you can make quick and easy lunches that are packed with protein and full of the right nutrients.

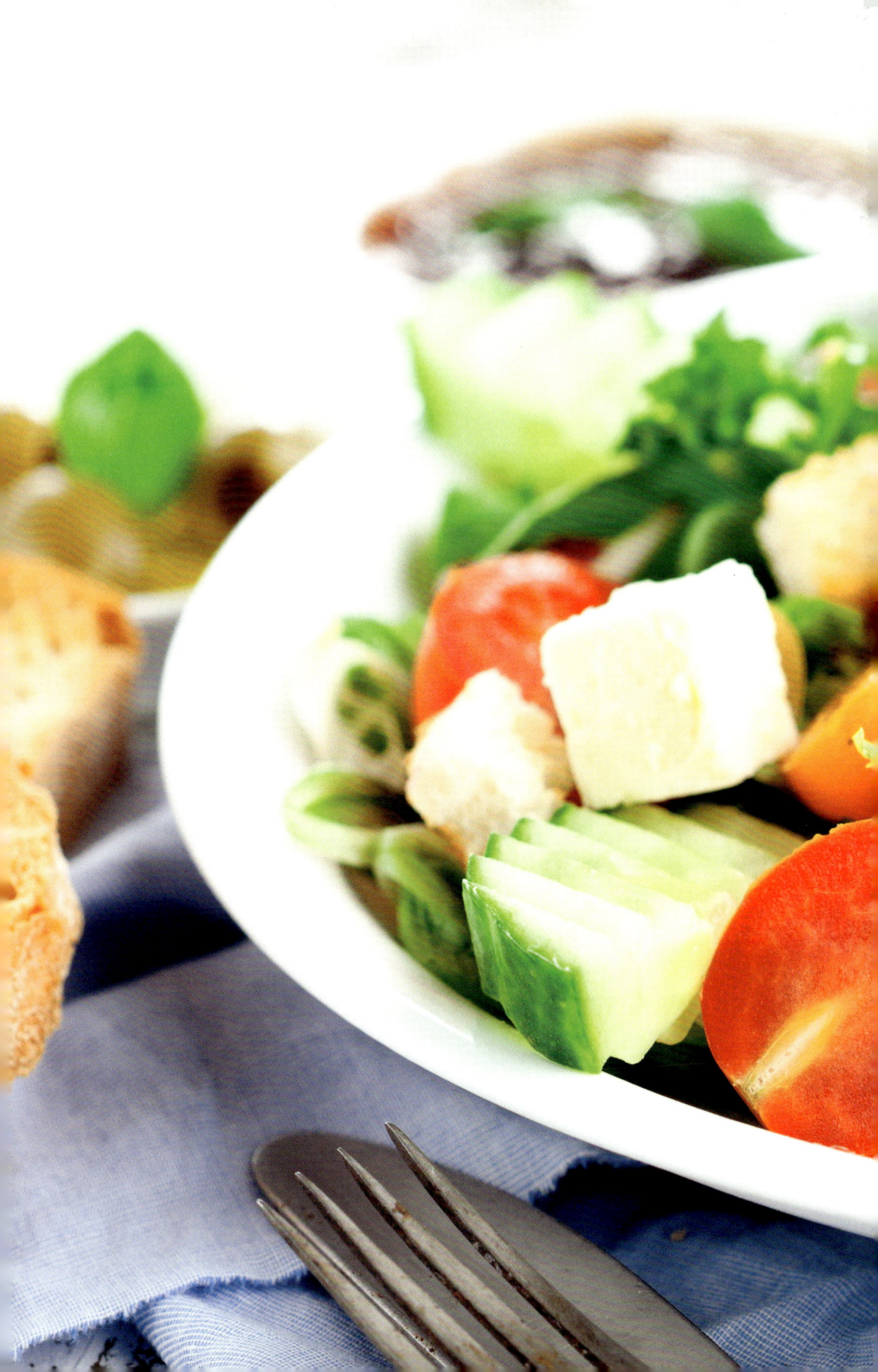

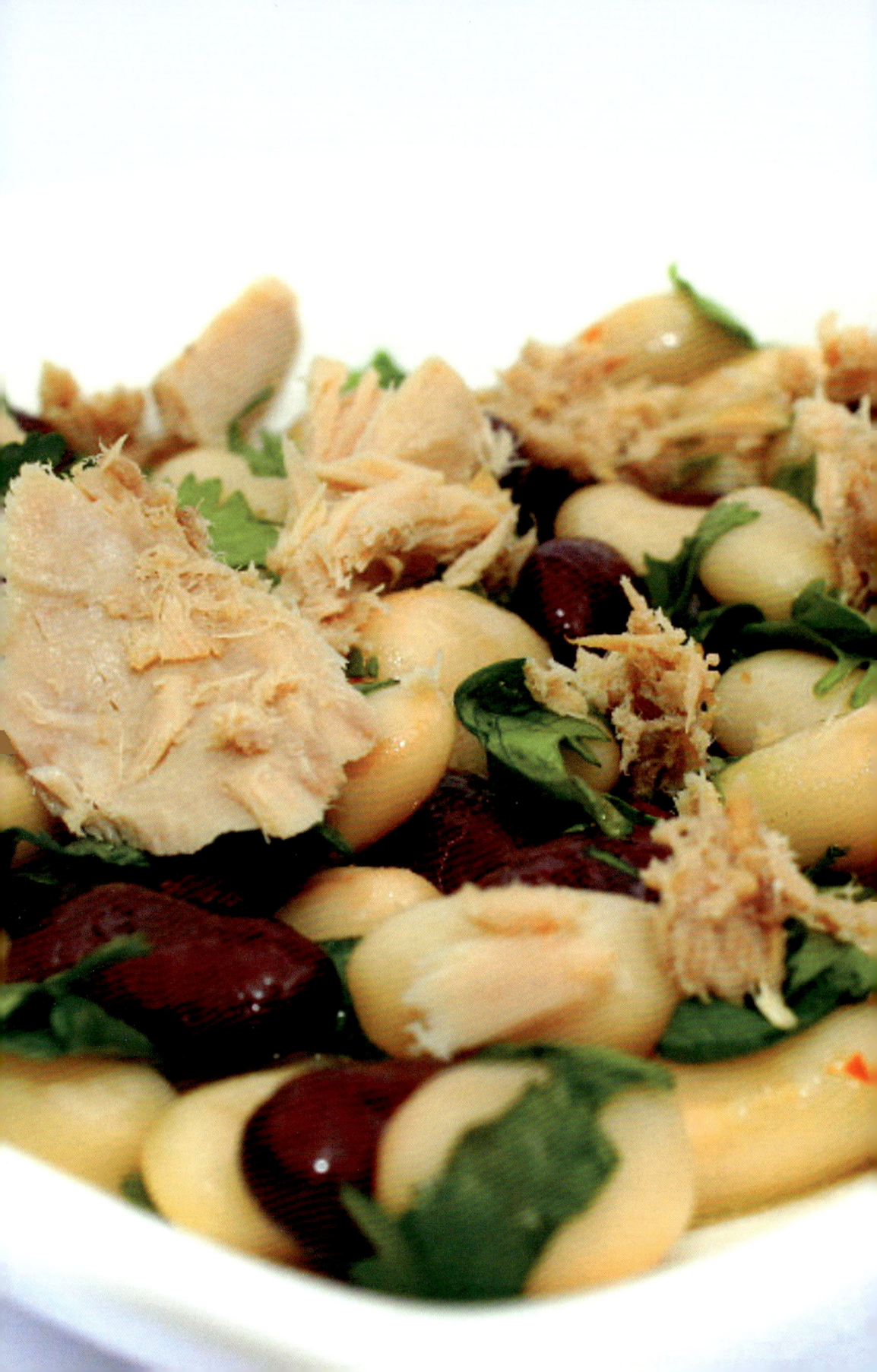

TIP

The real key to a good lunch is **planning**. Think ahead and make a little extra the night before, or if you have time in the morning, boil some eggs. You can also buy a pre-cooked chicken breast or a tin of tuna.

TUNA AND BEAN SALAD

INGREDIENTS

Small tin of tuna fish

150 ml of Butter beans

150 ml of Kidney beans

A handful of coriander, chopped

A drizzle of olive oil

Salt and pepper to taste

INSTRUCTIONS

Drain and rinse beans. Drain water from tuna.

Mix all the ingredients together and season to taste.

OPEN-FACED GRILLED HALLOUMI SANDWICH

INGREDIENTS

A few slices of halloumi

Splash of vinegar

1 egg

A handful of peas

10 small asparagus spears

1 slice of wholemeal bread, toasted

Pesto sauce

INSTRUCTIONS

Add the slices of halloumi to a frying pan and gently cook for about 3 minutes on each side.

Bring a pan of water to a boil. Add a splash of vinegar, turn the heat down to a simmer and crack your egg into it to gently poach.

Bring another pot of water to a boil. Add the peas first, allowing them to cook for 2 minutes. Add the asparagus and cook for a further 3 minutes.

Place the halloumi, egg, asparagus and peas on the toasted bread. Finish with a good helping of the pesto sauce.

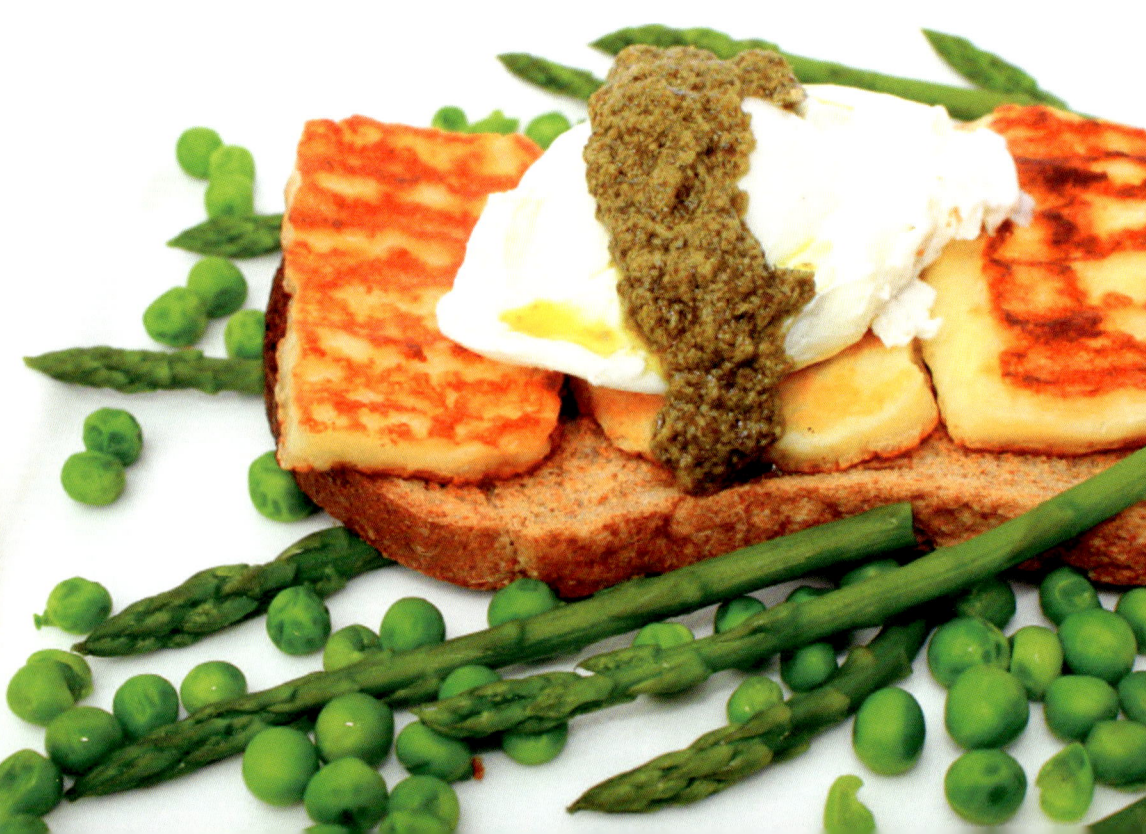

SUMMER SALAD

INGREDIENTS

- Rocket leaves
- Poached salmon
- Grapefruit, sliced
- Whole walnuts
- Feta cheese
- Chives
- Olive oil

INSTRUCTIONS

Place your rocket leaves onto a plate and scatter with pieces of poached salmon. Add grapefruit segments and walnuts. Sprinkle with feta cheese and chives.

Drizzle with a small amount of olive oil to finish.

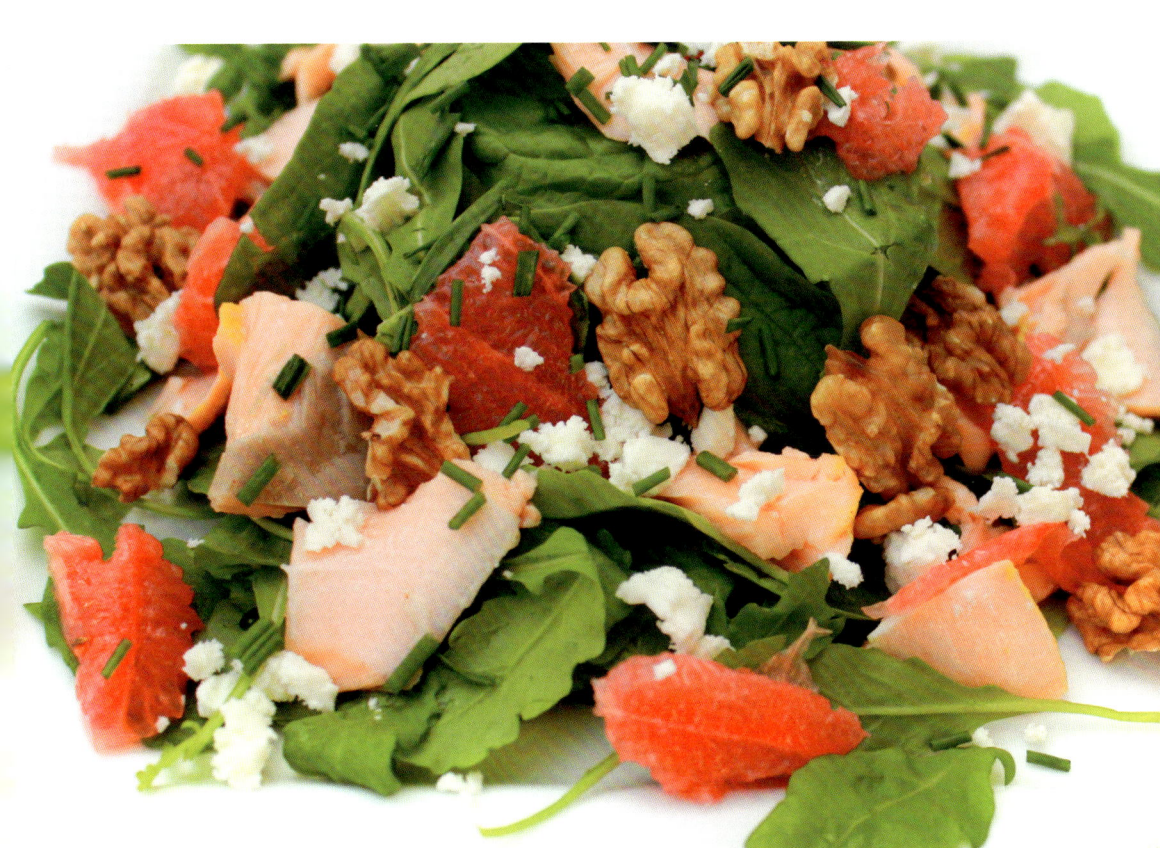

ROASTED RED PEPPER AND TOMATO SOUP

INGREDIENTS

- 2 red bell peppers
- A handful of cherry tomatoes
- 2 cloves of garlic
- 1 small onion, chopped
- Half of a red chilli
- A good splash of basil oil
- A small squirt of tomato purée
- A pinch of mixed herbs
- 500ml of water
- 1 cube of vegetable stock
- Spring onions for garnish

INSTRUCTIONS

Preheat oven to 180° C. Add the vegetables, garlic and chili to a roasting dish, drizzle with basil oil, and roast for about 40 minutes until soft.

Allow to cool, then transfer to a blender. Add tomato purée and mixed herbs and blitz for 30 seconds, until you have a soft pulp.

In a saucepan, dissolve the cube of vegetable stock in 500ml of water and add the puréed vegetable mixture. Gently simmer to your desired temperature.

Garnish with spring onion and enjoy.

TIP

THIS IS A GREAT ONE TO DO AT THE WEEKEND. WHY NOT MAKE A BIG BATCH AND FREEZE IT FOR THE WEEK AHEAD?

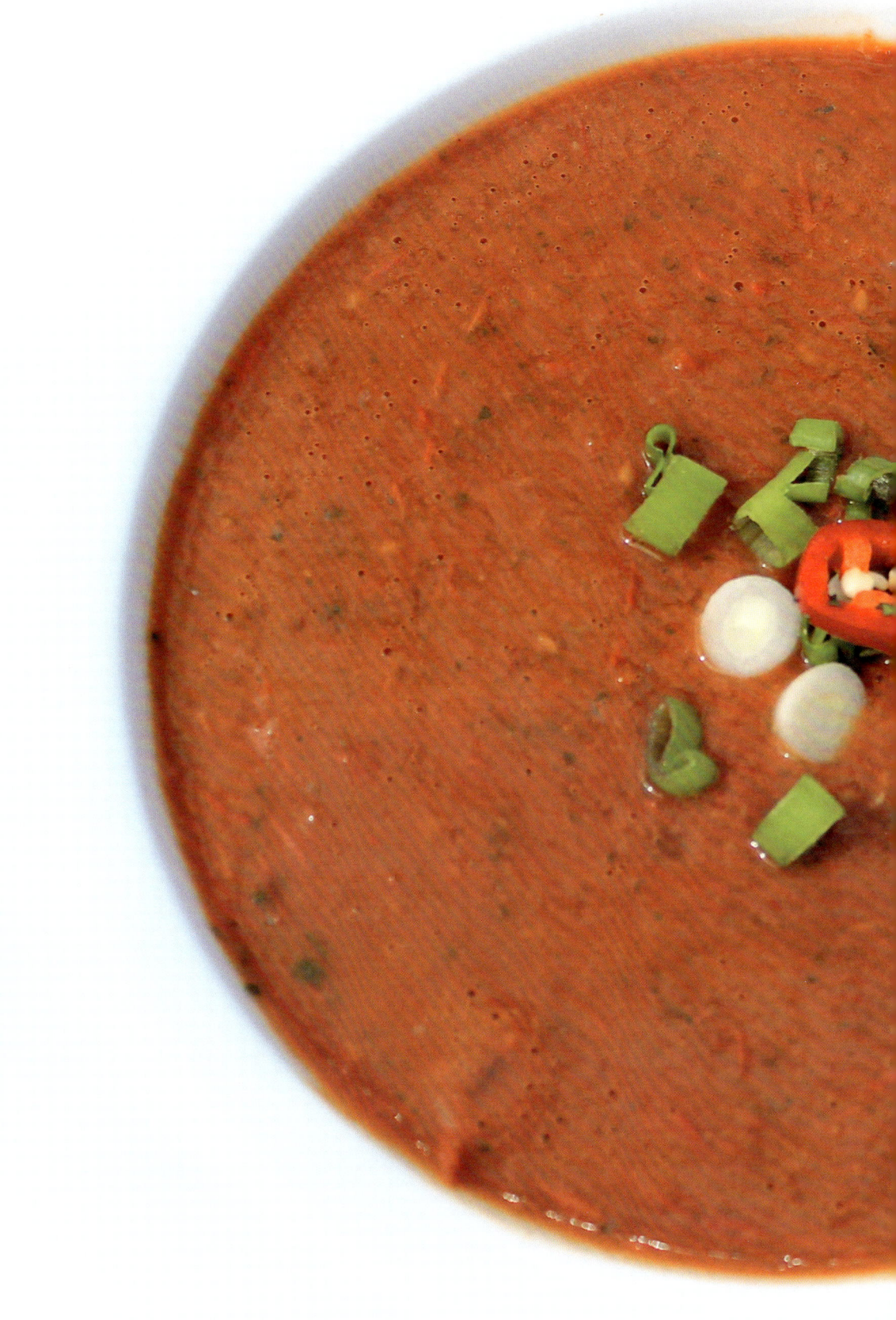

PEA AND ROCKET SOUP

INGREDIENTS

A drizzle of olive oil

1 small onion, diced

1 very large handful of rocket leaves

1 large handful of peas

500 ml of vegetable stock

Greek yoghurt

INSTRUCTIONS

In a large saucepan, heat the olive oil and cook the onion until soft.

Pour in the stock and cook for around 8 minutes.

Add the peas and rocket, bring to a boil and cook for around 4 minutes until all is tender. Remove from heat and allow to cool down.

Carefully pour into a blender and give it a quick blitz till you have a nice texture. Return to the pan and gently reheat.

Serve with a spoonful of Greek yoghurt.

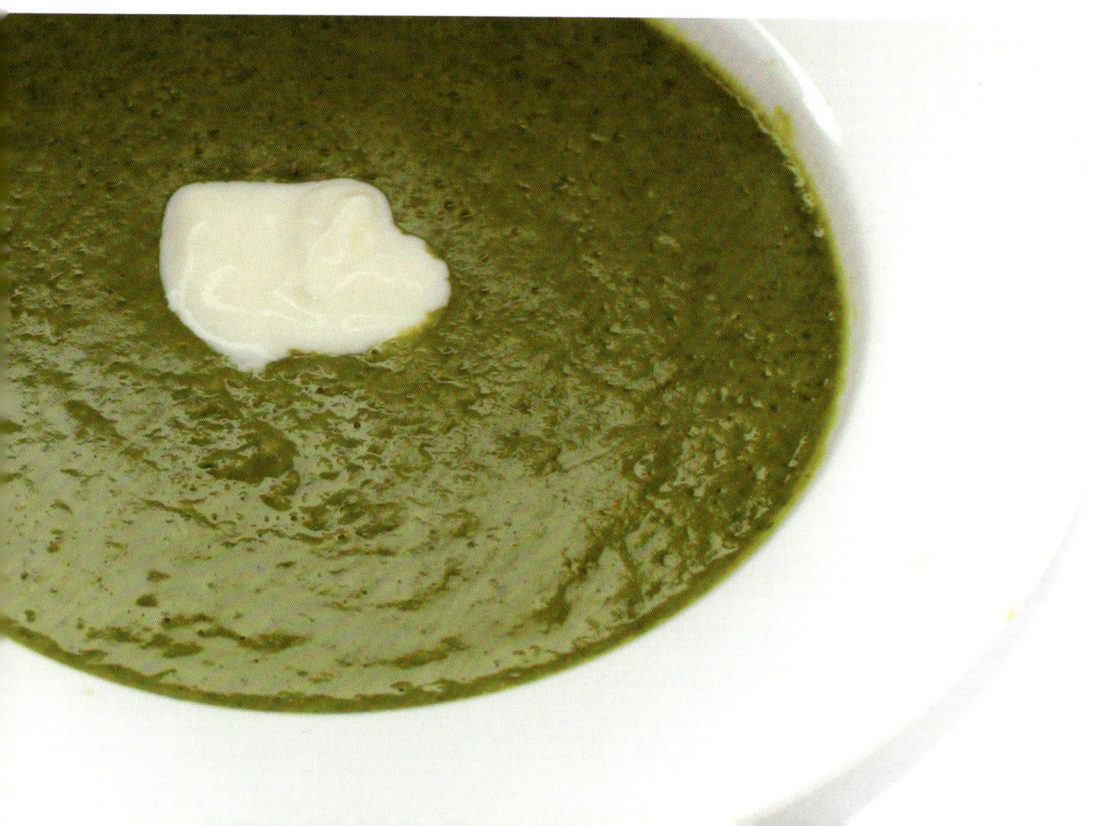

CHICKEN AND APPLE SALAD

INGREDIENTS

A few slices of pre-cooked chicken, shredded

1 apple, chopped

1 handful of sugar snap peas

A handful of walnuts

Natural yoghurt

Pomegranate seeds

Chives

INSTRUCTIONS

Mix all of the ingredients together with a few spoonfuls of yoghurt.

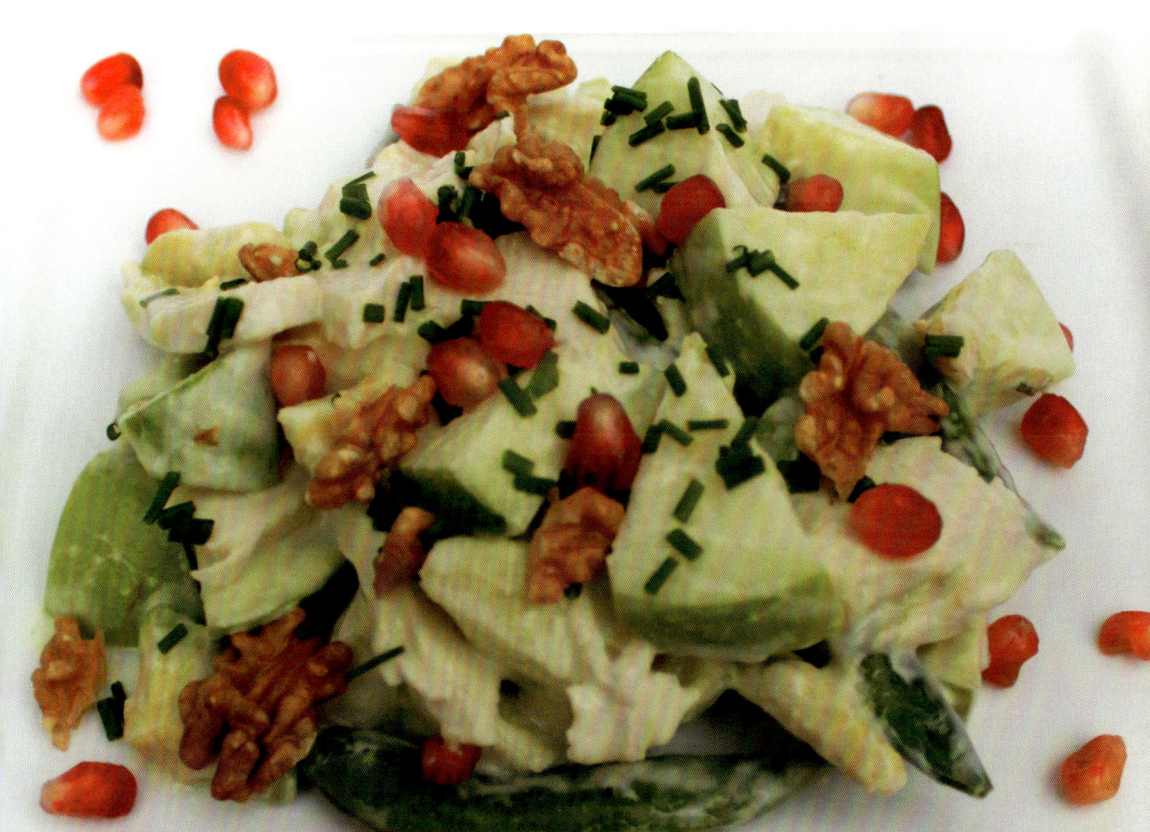

TUNA BOAT

INGREDIENTS

1 small tin of tuna

2 spring onions, chopped

Red pepper, chopped

Crème fraiche

2 leaves of romaine lettuce, washed

INSTRUCTIONS

Mix all of the ingredients together with a couple of spoon of crème fraiche. Spoon into the lettuce leaves to serve.

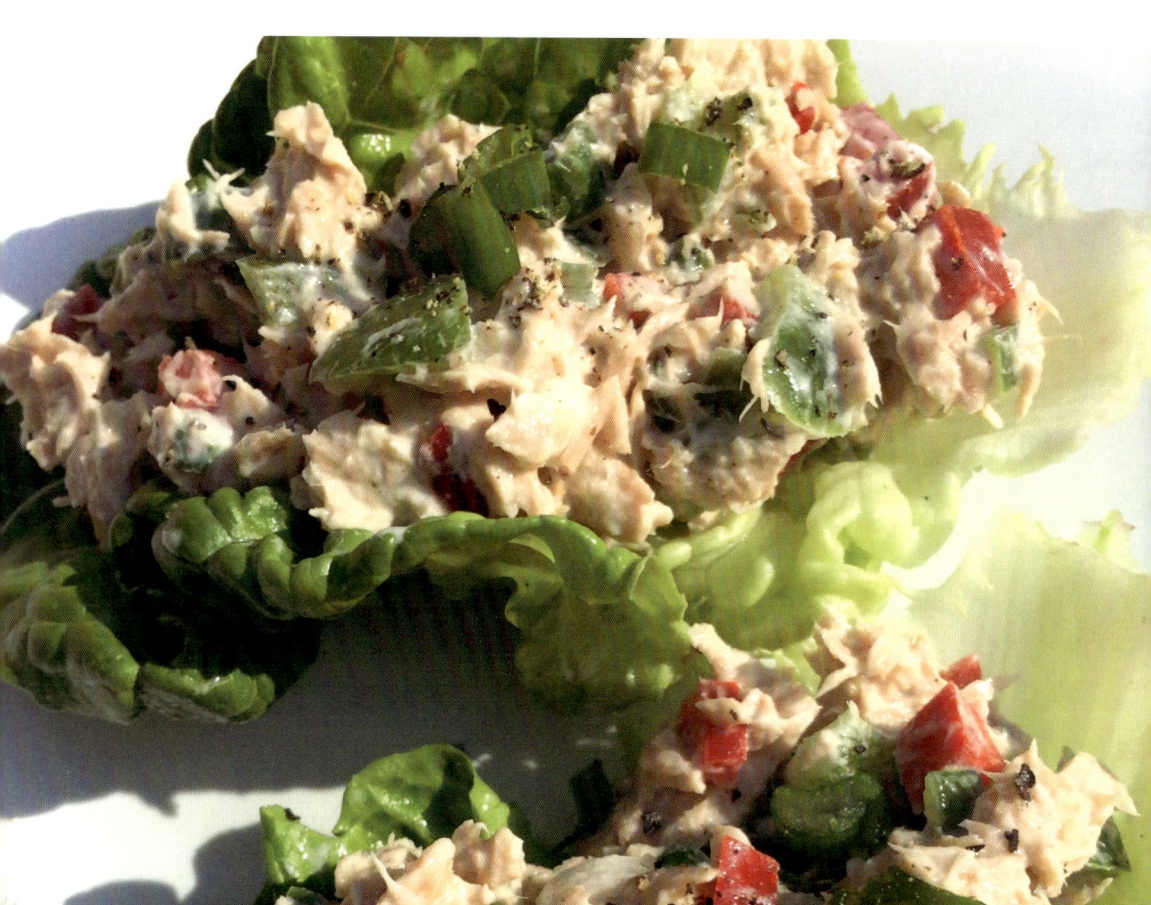

TOMATO AND MOZZARELLA STACK

INGREDIENTS

A handful of asparagus

2 beef tomatoes, sliced

4 slices of Mozzarella, sliced

Salt and pepper to taste

Balsamic oil

Rocket leaves

INSTRUCTIONS

Bring a small saucepan of water to a boil. Add the asparagus and simmer for 3 minutes. Drain, rinse in cold water and set aside to cool.

Carefully stack the tomato and mozzarella slices.

Season with salt and pepper and drizzle with balsamic oil. Scatter some rocket leaves to dress.

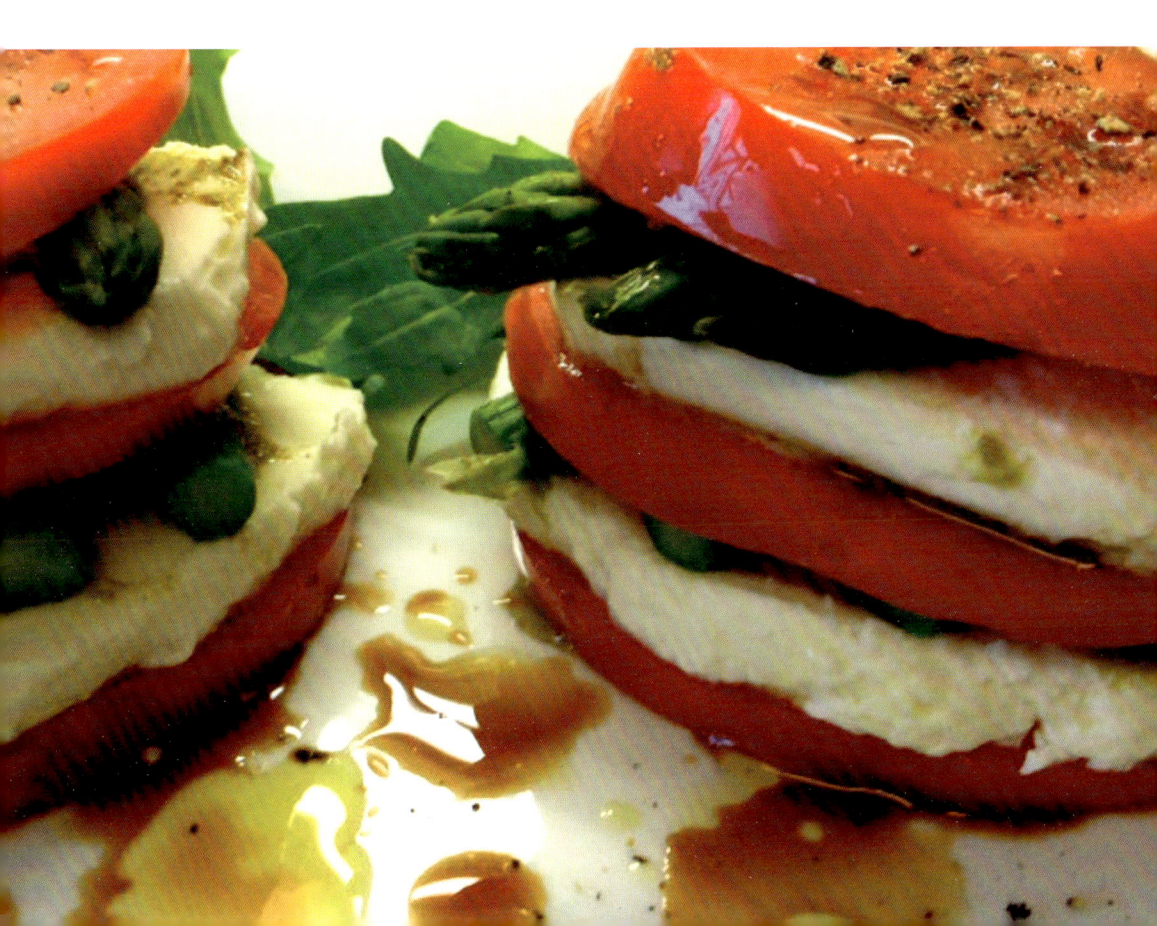

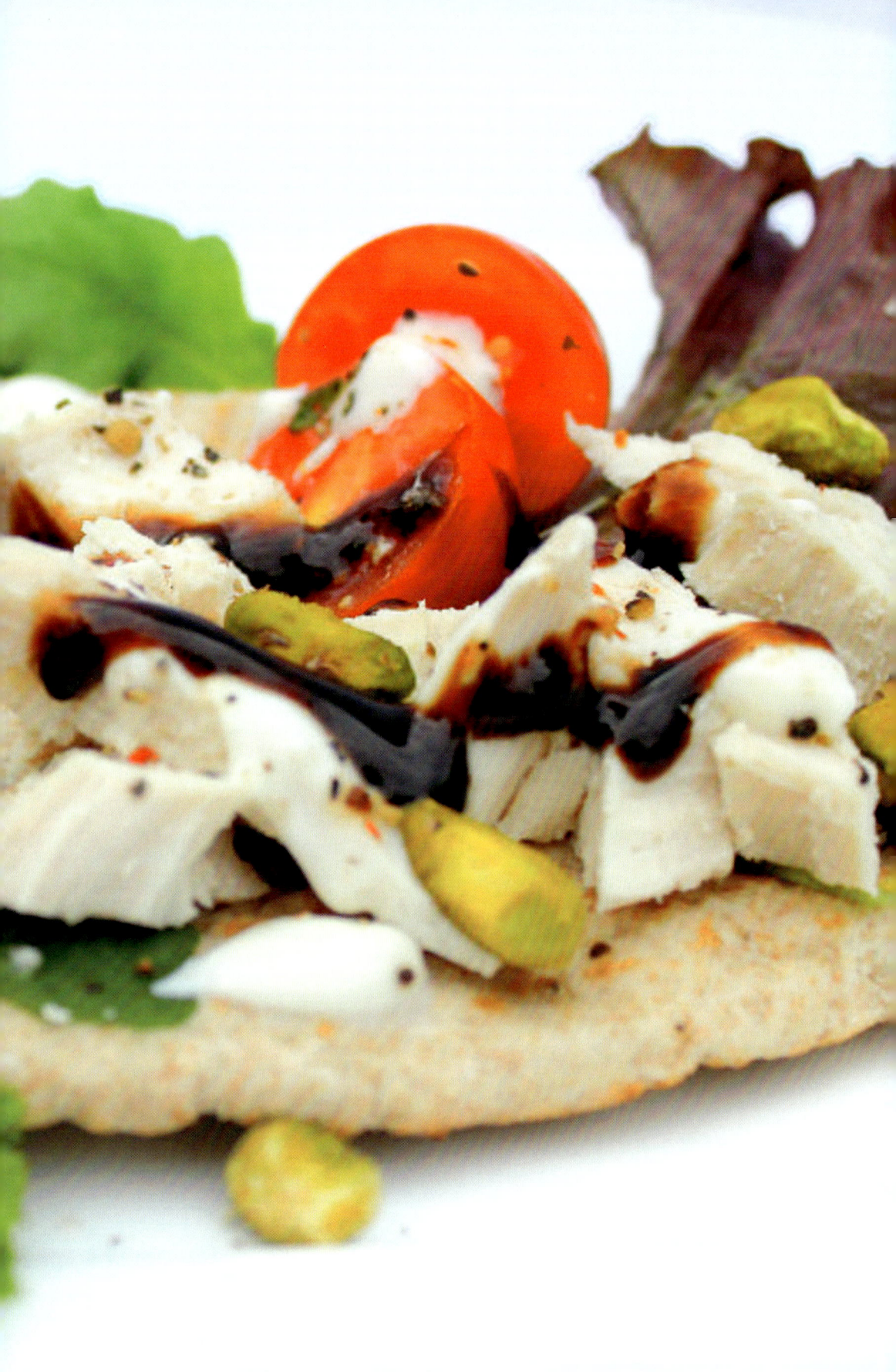

OPEN-FACED CHICKEN PITTA

INGREDIENTS

1 wholemeal pitta

1 small chicken breast, cooked and shredded

1 small tomato, sliced

Balsamic glaze

Pistachio nuts

Salt and pepper to taste

INSTRUCTIONS

Warm the pitta. Scatter the shredded chicken over the pitta and top with sliced tomato.

Drizzle with balsamic glaze. Add a few pistachio nuts and season to taste.

TIP

THIS IS A GREAT ONE TO DO AT YOUR OFFICE; ALL YOU NEED IS A TOASTER TO WARM THE PITTA.

TOMATO AND NECTARINE SALAD

INGREDIENTS

A handful of mixed salad leaves

1 nectarine, peeled and sliced

A handful of cherry tomatoes, halved

A small portion of Feta cheese, crumbled

Chives, chopped

Olive oil

INSTRUCTIONS

Add the mixed salad leaves, nectarine, tomatoes and feta to a bowl.

Drizzle with olive oil and dress with chives.

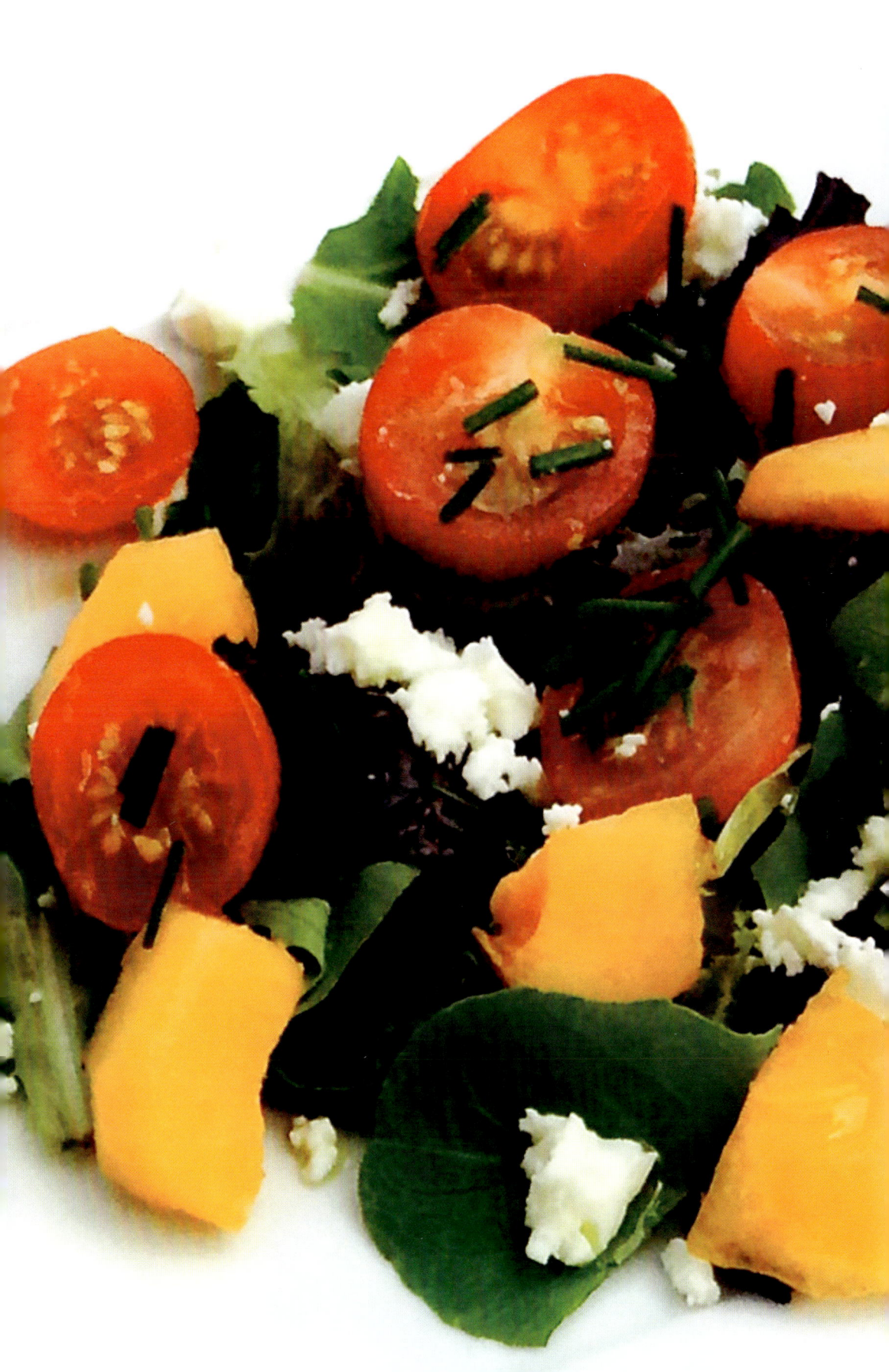

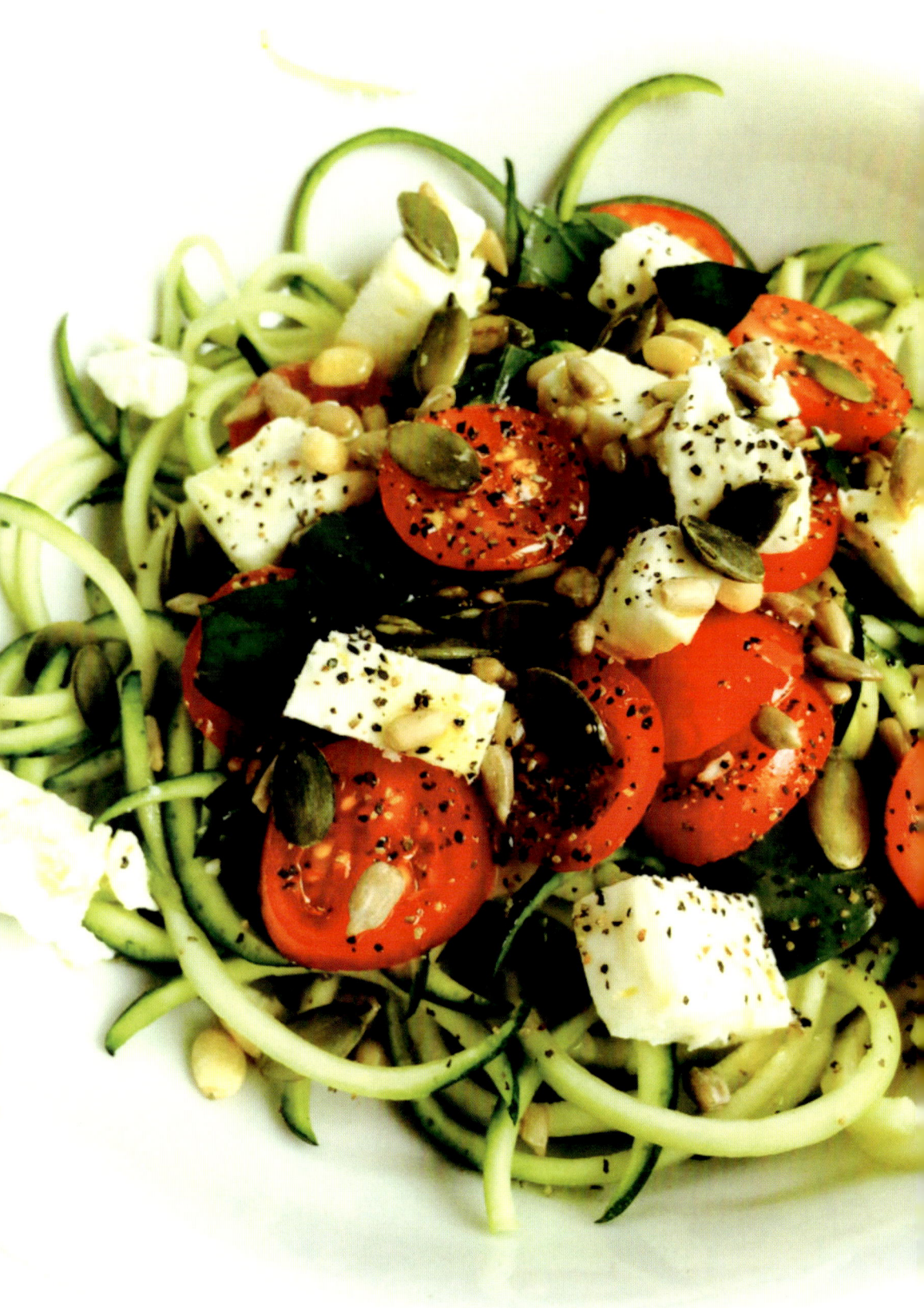

ZUCCHINI PASTA

INGREDIENTS

1 small zucchini, spiralised into pasta ribbons

2 tsps. of Green pesto sauce

4 cherry tomatoes

Feta cheese, crumbled

A handful of mixed salad seeds

Fresh basil leaves

Olive oil

Salt and pepper to taste

INSTRUCTIONS

Toss the pesto sauce with the spiralised zucchini. Add the tomatoes, feta and salad seeds.

Dress with shredded basil leaves and olive oil and season to taste.

TIP

A SPIRALISER IS A HAND-HELD TOOL THAT VERY SIMPLY TURNS A ZUCCHINI INTO PASTA NOODLES.

GRILLED HALLOUMI AND ASPARAGUS

INGREDIENTS

A good handful of asparagus

1 slice of halloumi

Tomatoes

Pomegranate seeds

Poppy seeds

INSTRUCTIONS

Heat a griddle pan, add slice of halloumi and cook for around 3 minutes on each side.

Bring a pot of water to a boil, add the asparagus and cook for around 3 minutes.

Add the asparagus to your plate, lay the halloumi over the asparagus and dress with tomato and pomegranate seeds. Finish with a sprinkle of poppy seeds.

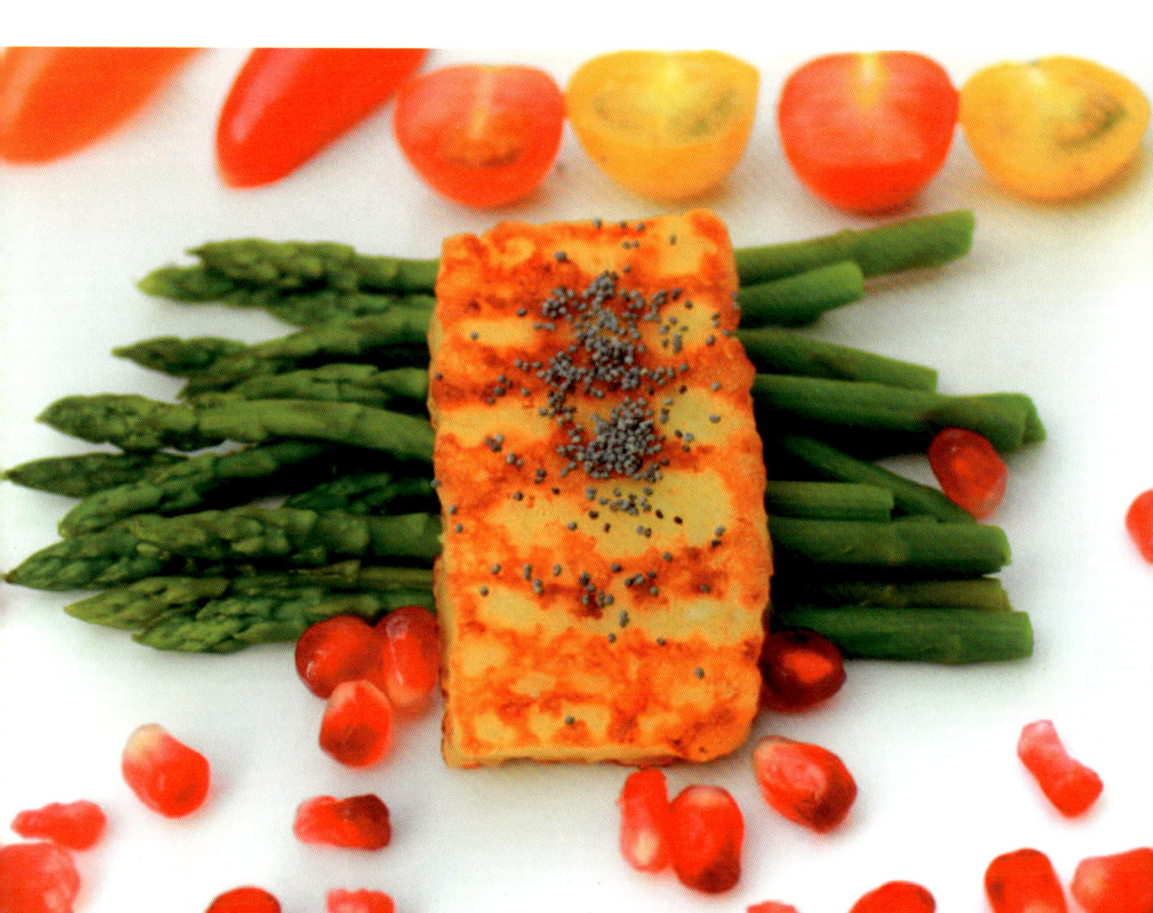

Lunch

TORTILLA WRAP

INGREDIENTS

1 wholemeal tortilla

Half of an avocado, sliced

1 boiled egg, sliced

1 slice of smoked salmon

Pomegranate

Rocket leaves

INSTRUCTIONS

Place all of the ingredients in the middle of the tortilla. Carefully fold each side and one end. Dress with pomegranate and rocket leaves.

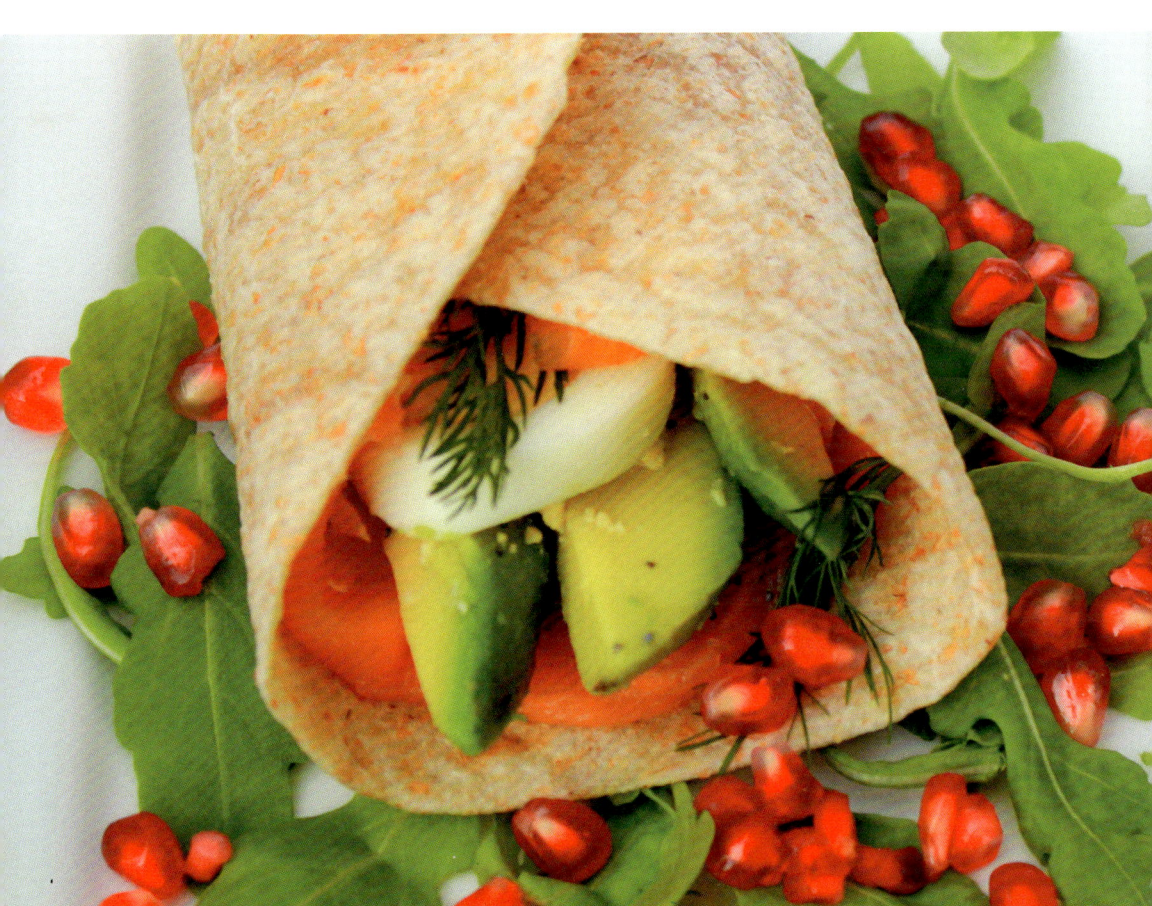

9 DINNER

Eating a healthy dinner has a number of essential functions. As it leads up to the time your body needs to repair itself from your daily routine, you need to make the right choices. Skipping dinner results in low levels of insulin and blood sugar in your body. This causes your body to go into starvation mode and use up all the other energy reserves. As a result, your body will not get the necessary nutrition it needs on a regular basis.

A healthy dinner should consist of protein and a small portion of good carbohydrate. Having a healthy meal before you sleep can actually help you sleep better and lose weight.

TIP

- Preparation is the key to a healthy dinner.

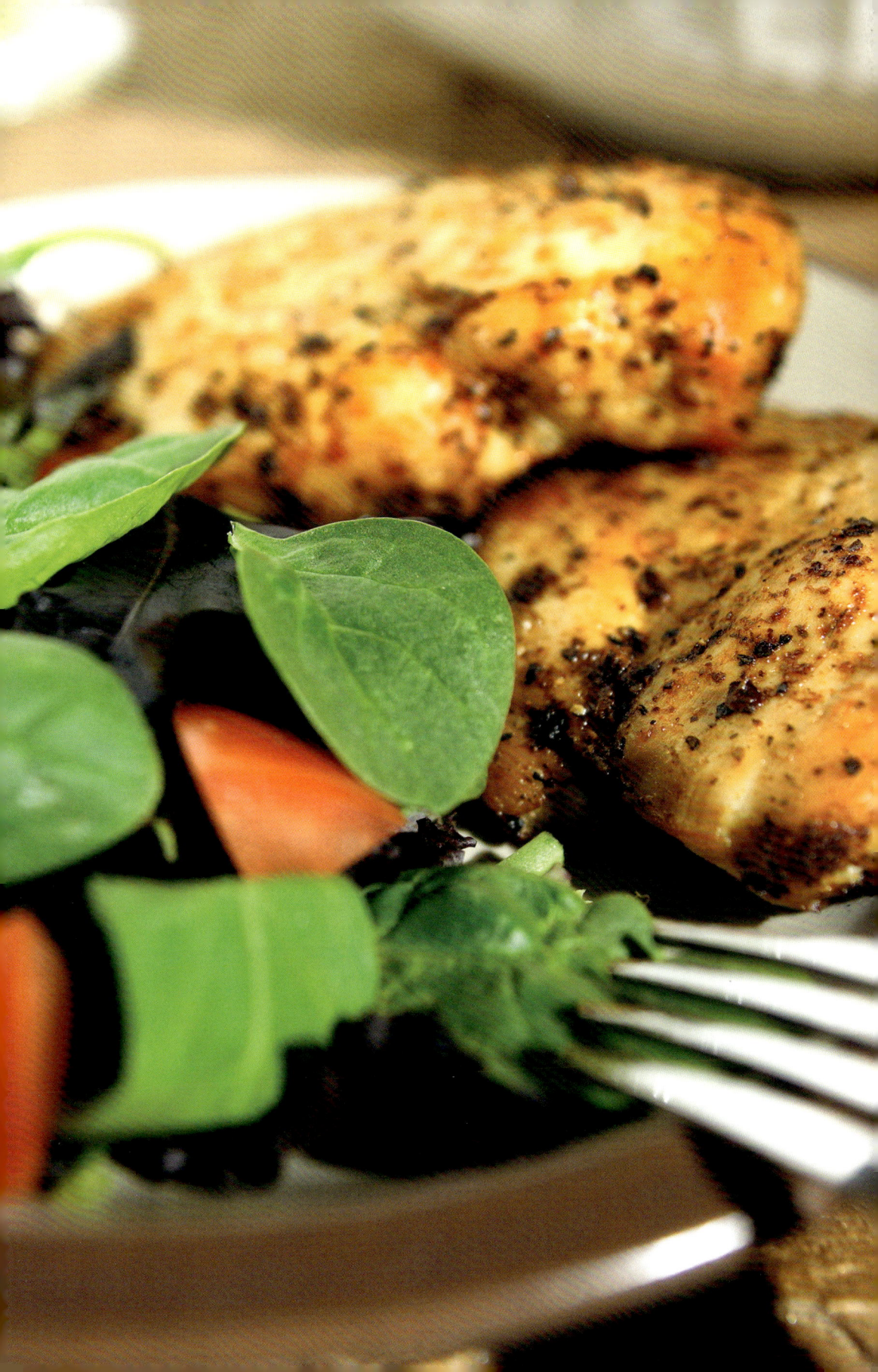

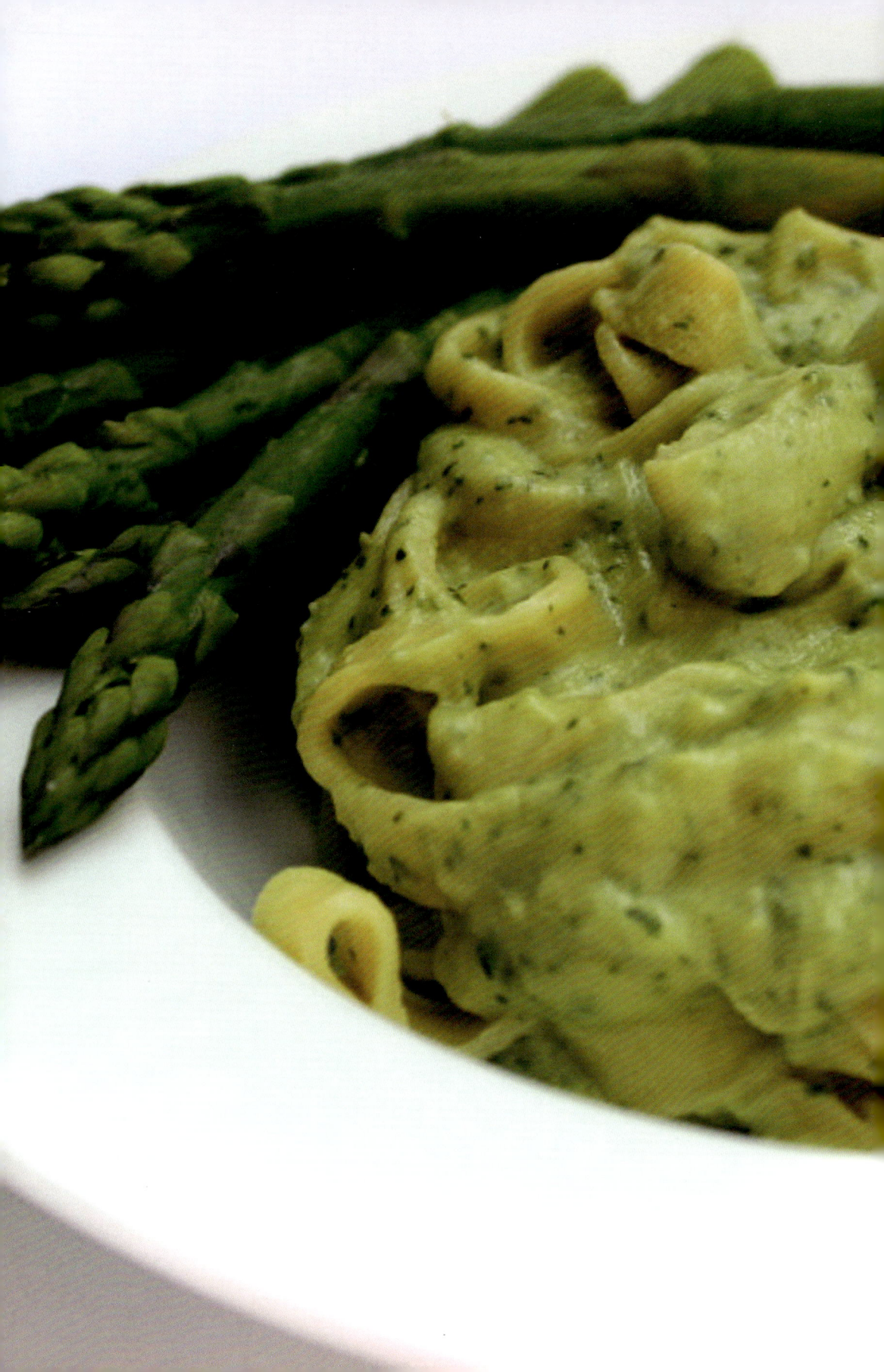

BASIL AND AVOCADO PASTA

INGREDIENTS

1 avocado, chopped

A good handful of fresh basil, chopped

1 cup of milk

A handful of asparagus

A portion of fresh wholemeal tagliatelle

Salt and pepper to taste

INSTRUCTIONS

Put the avocado and basil into a blender and give a quick blitz. This should now be a thick paste. Slowly add the milk, and blitz until you get a good consistency of sauce. Pour the sauce into a small saucepan and heat.

Bring a pot of water to a boil and add the tagliatelle and cook for 3 minutes.

Bring a second pot of water to a boil, add asparagus and cook asparagus for 3 minutes.

When both are cooked, mix together with the warmed sauce and season to taste.

COD WITH COCONUT AND DILL

INGREDIENTS

1 medium sized Cod fillet

A handful of dill finely chopped

300ml of coconut milk

A handful of asparagus

INSTRUCTIONS

Place the cod in a griddle pan with the dill and cover with the coconut milk. Gently simmer for about 10 minutes on a low heat.

Bring a pot of water to a boil and cook the asparagus for three minutes. Drain, and serve with the cod. Season to taste.

TIP

BE SURE NOT TO OVERCOOK THE ASPARAGUS, AS YOU WILL TAKE OUT ALL OF THE GOODNESS THAT THE ASPARAGUS HAS TO OFFER.

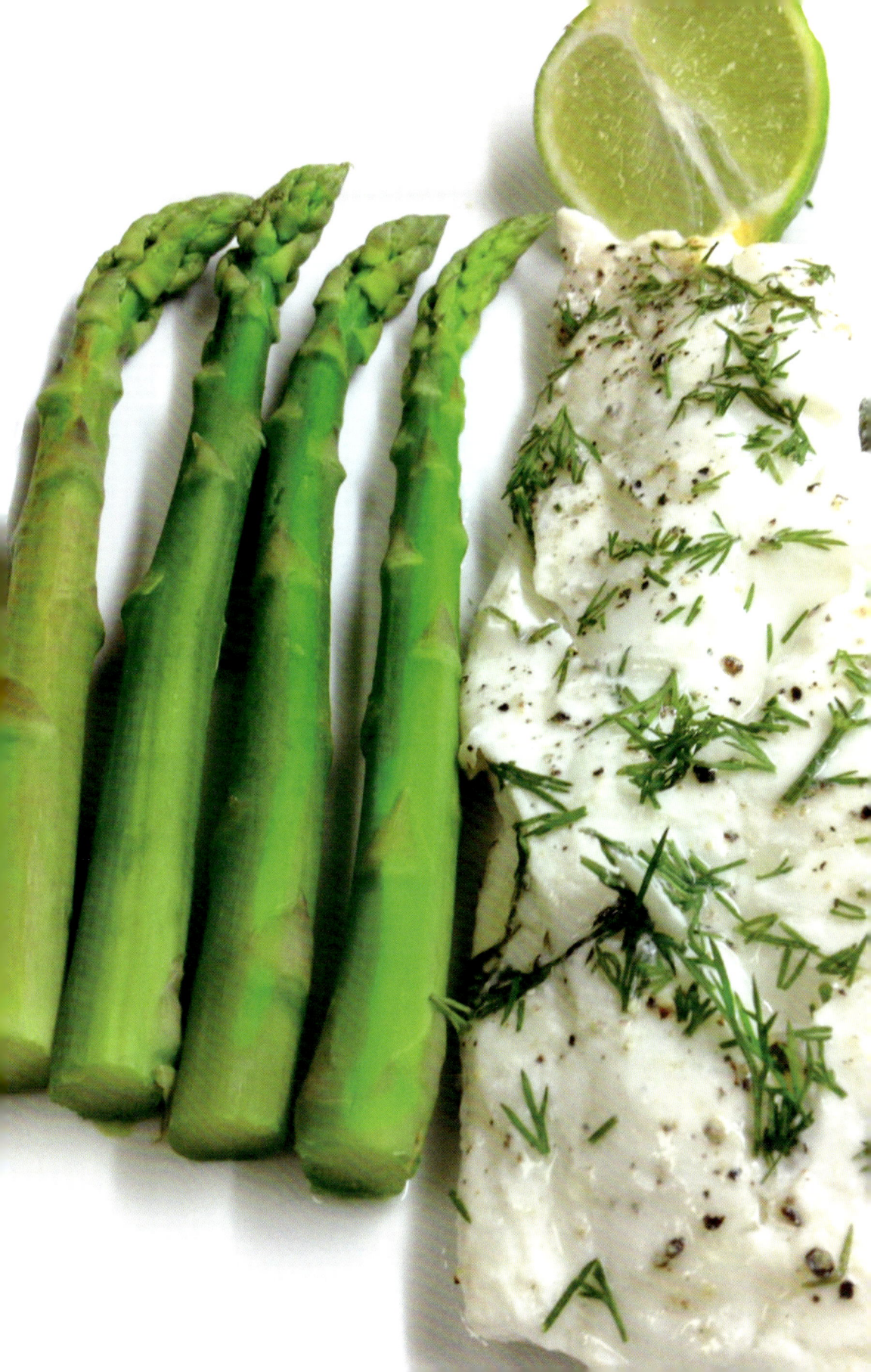

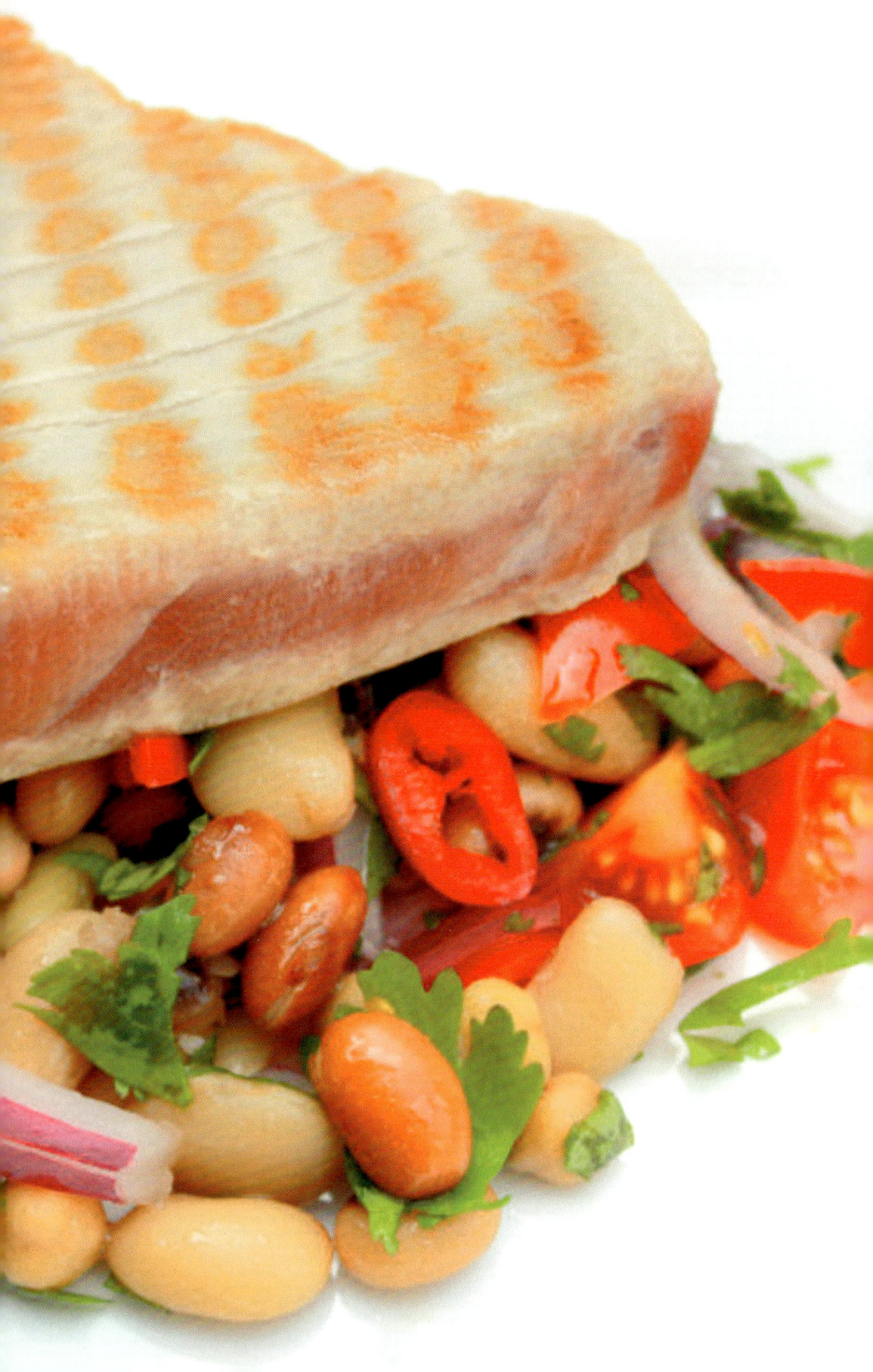

TUNA AND BEAN SALSA

INGREDIENTS

150g of Butter beans

150g of Haricot beans

1 small red onion, diced

1 medium tomato, diced

1 small red chilli, diced

1 small handful of coriander, chopped

Olive oil

1 medium sized tuna steak

Salt and pepper to taste

INSTRUCTIONS

Combine the beans, onion, tomato, chilli and coriander in a bowl, and add a drizzle of Olive oil.

Heat a griddle pan to a high heat, and sear the tuna steak for 2 minutes on each side, keeping it rare in the middle.

Spoon the salsa mix onto your plate, and add the tuna on top. Season with salt and black pepper to taste.

AVOCADO SCALLOPS

INGREDIENTS

6 scallops

1 avocado

Small piece of feta cheese

Juice of a lime

A handful of asparagus

INSTRUCTIONS

In a bowl, mash the avocado, feta and half of the lime juice.

Bring a pot of water to a boil. Drop the asparagus in the boiling water and cook for 2 minutes. Drain.

Heat a griddle pan to medium heat. Place the scallops in the griddle pan and cook for 2 minute on each side.

Place the asparagus and scallops on your plate and spoon a small amount of the avocado mixture onto each scallop.

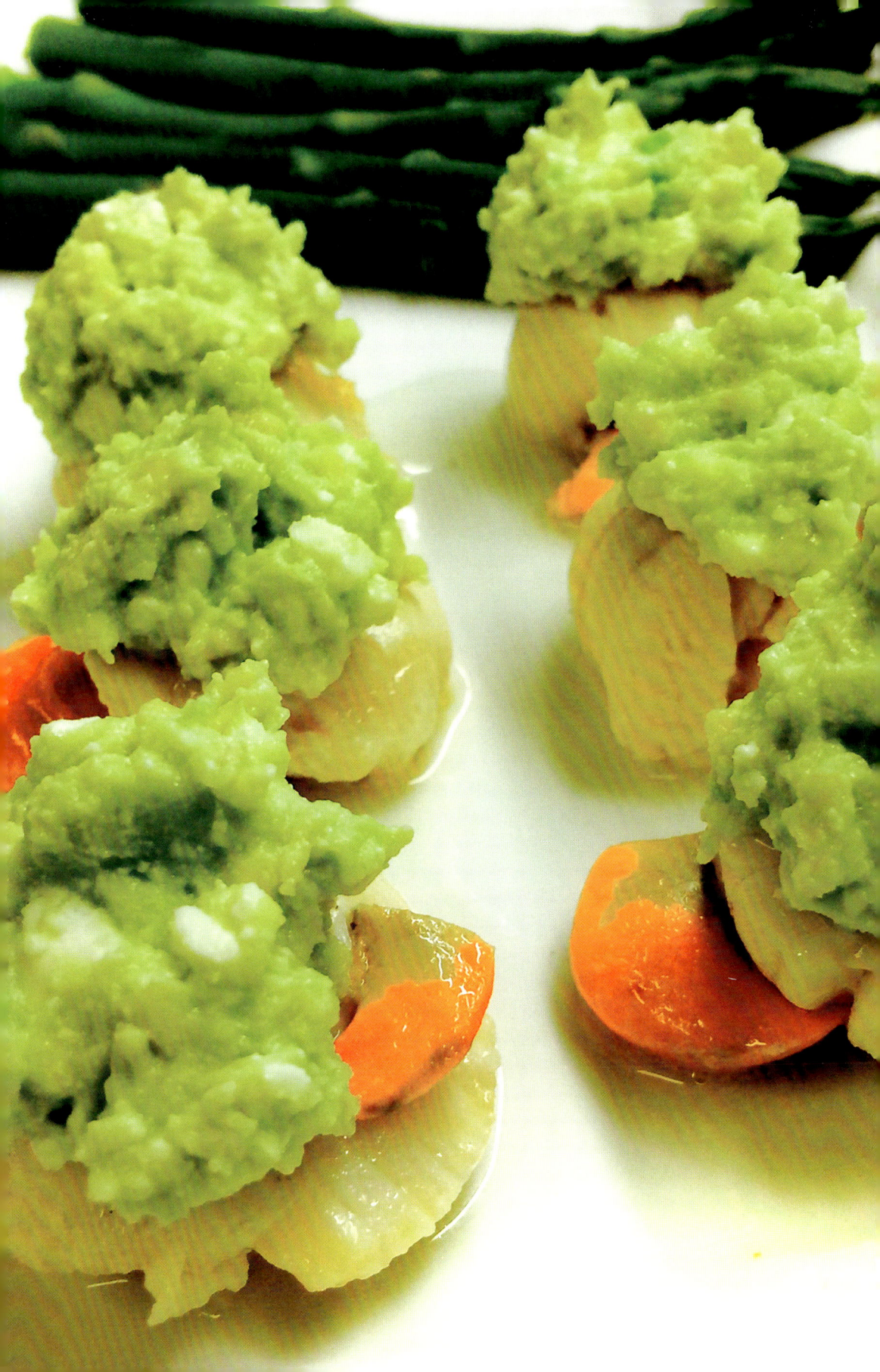

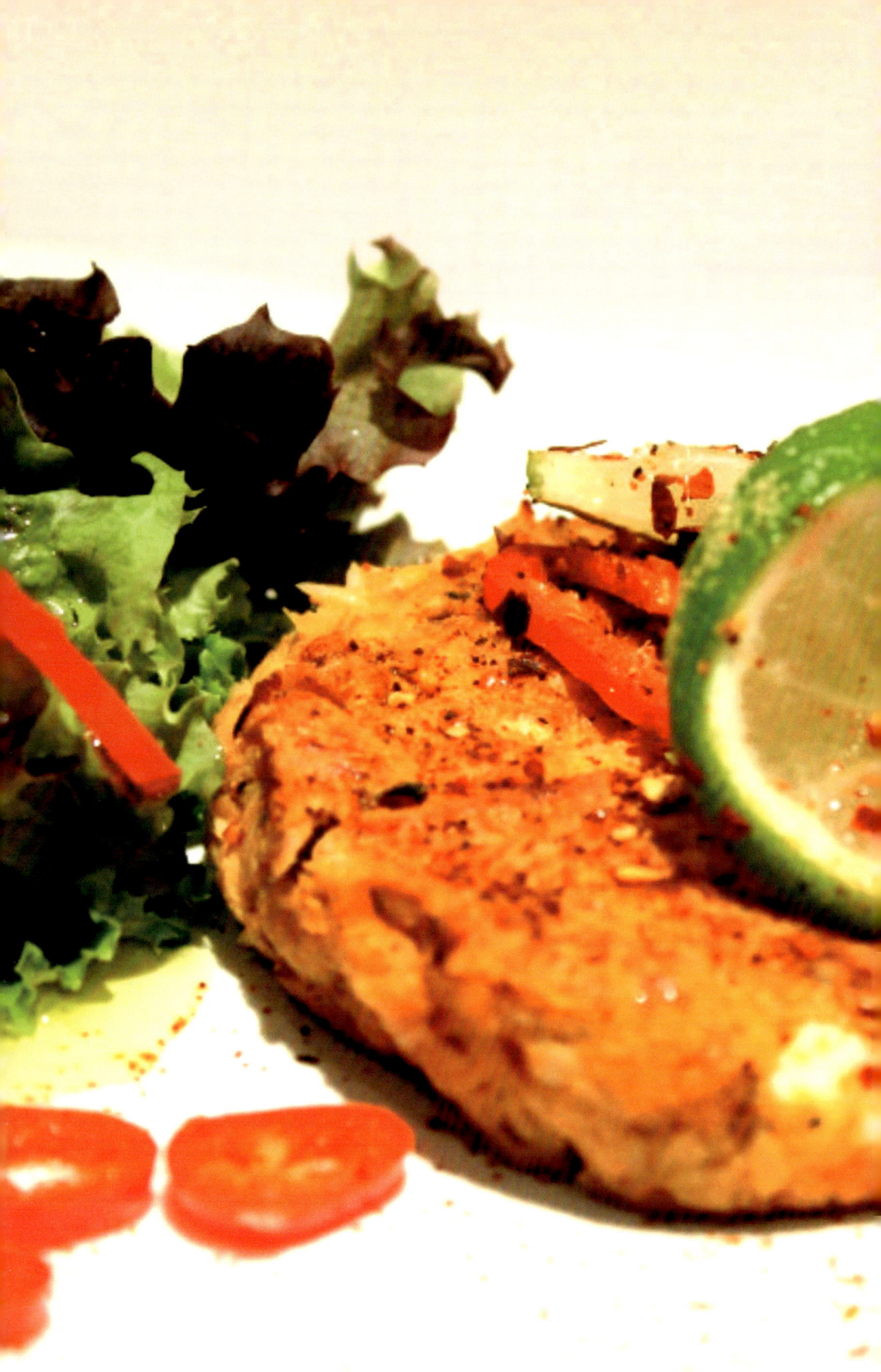

SALMON CAKE

INGREDIENTS

1 sweet potato, peeled and diced

1 small piece of salmon

Wholemeal breadcrumbs

A pinch of paprika

Juice from half of a lime

A pinch of chili flakes

A small portion of Feta cheese, crumbled

Olive oil

INSTRUCTIONS

Bring a pot of water to a boil and cook the diced sweet potato for 10-12 minutes, until tender. Drain, mash and set aside.

Lightly brush the Salmon with Olive oil and grill for 10 minutes.

Flake the salmon into the sweet potato, and add the breadcrumbs, paprika, lime juice, chili flakes and feta cheese.

Mould into a cake, and pan-fry with a drizzle of Olive oil for about 5 minutes on each side.

Serve with a side salad of your choice.

TIP

TOAST AND CRUMBLE ONE SLICE OF BROWN BREAD TO MAKE YOUR OWN WHOLEMEAL BREADCRUMBS.

CRAB LINGUINE

INGREDIENTS

Linguini

Crab meat

1 garlic clove

Red pepper,

Spring onion

Juice of a lemon

INSTRUCTIONS

Heat a griddle pan and lightly fry the garlic. Set aside.

Gently mix the crab meat, red pepper, spring onion together in a bowl with half of the lemon juice.

Bring a large pot of water to a boil, add the linguini and cook until tender.

Once the linguini is cooked, drain and place in the griddle pan with the garlic on a low heat. Add the rest of the mixture and gently stir for around 3 minutes. Place in a pasta bowl to serve.

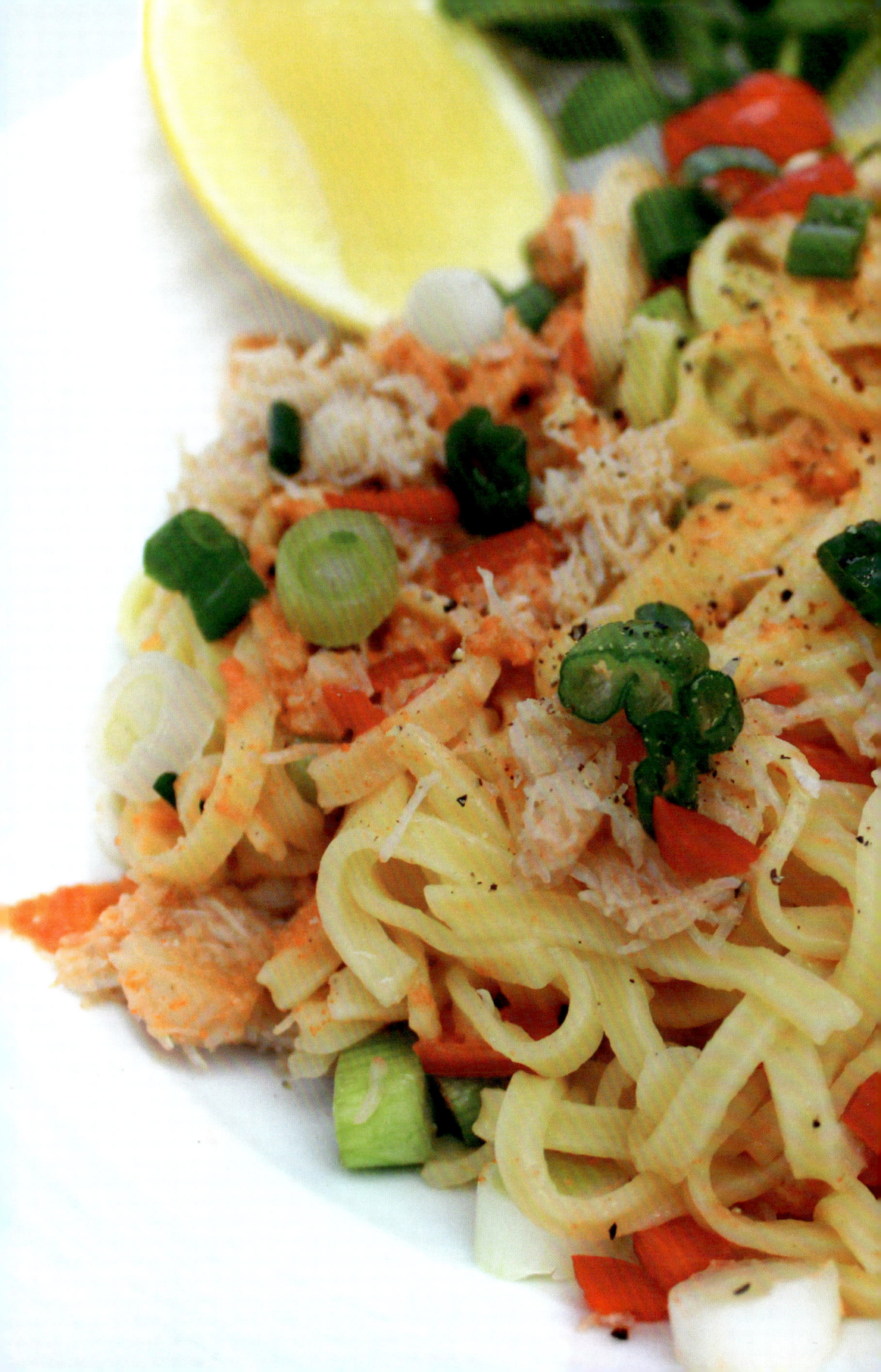

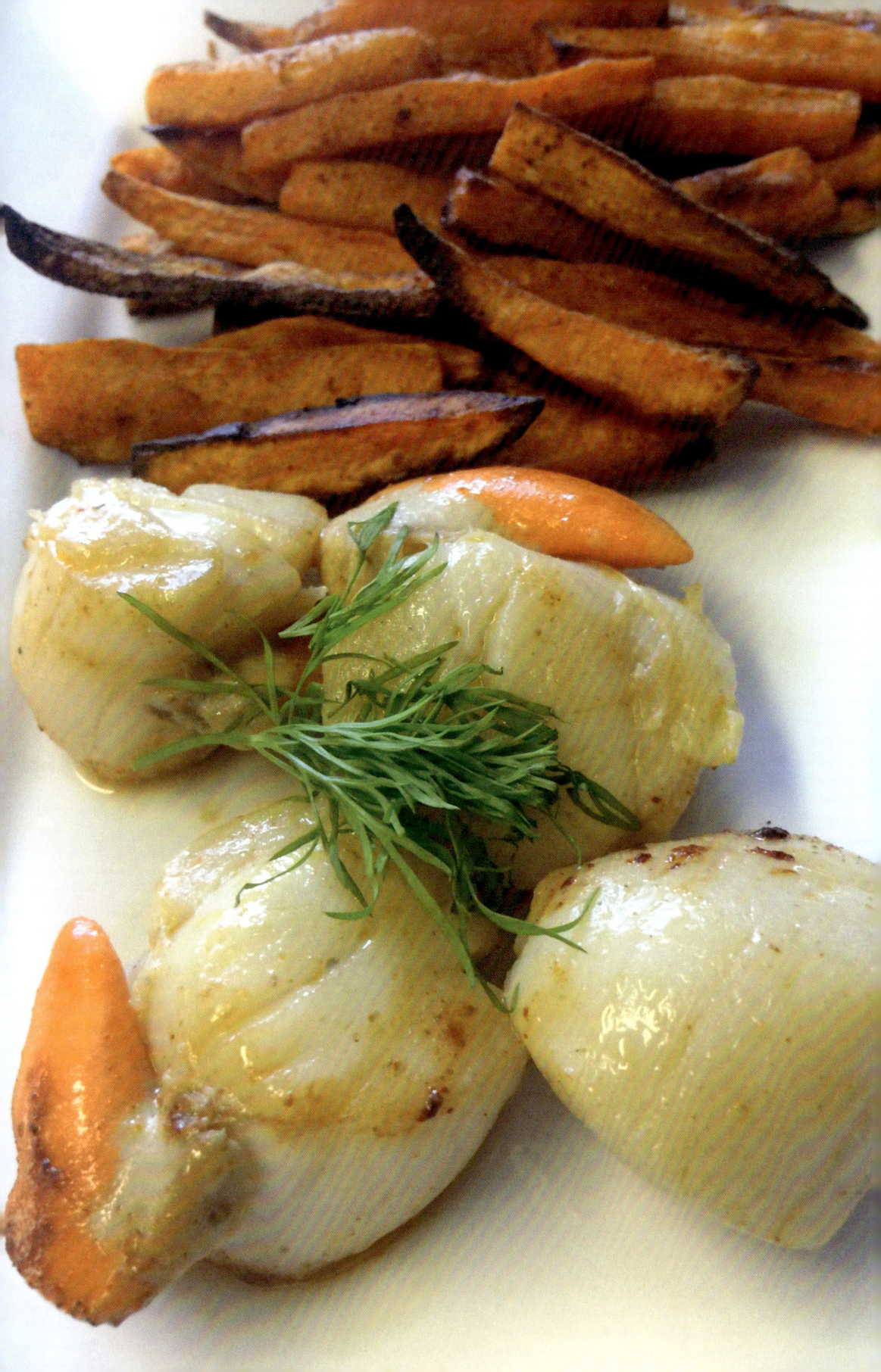

SCALLOPS AND SWEET POTATO FRIES

INGREDIENTS

4-6 scallops

1 sweet potato, peeled and chopped into bite-sized pieces

INSTRUCTIONS

Preheat oven to 200° C Place sweet potato pieces on a baking tray and bake for about 25 minutes until they are nicely brown, turning occasionally.

Heat a griddle pan and cook the scallops for two minutes on each side.

COD WITH BAKED CHERRY TOMATOES

INGREDIENTS

1 small piece of Cod

A good helping of sweet cherry tomatoes

INSTRUCTIONS

Preheat oven to 180° C. Place the cod and cherry tomatoes together on a baking pan and cook for 12 minutes.

Gently arrange onto your plate to serve

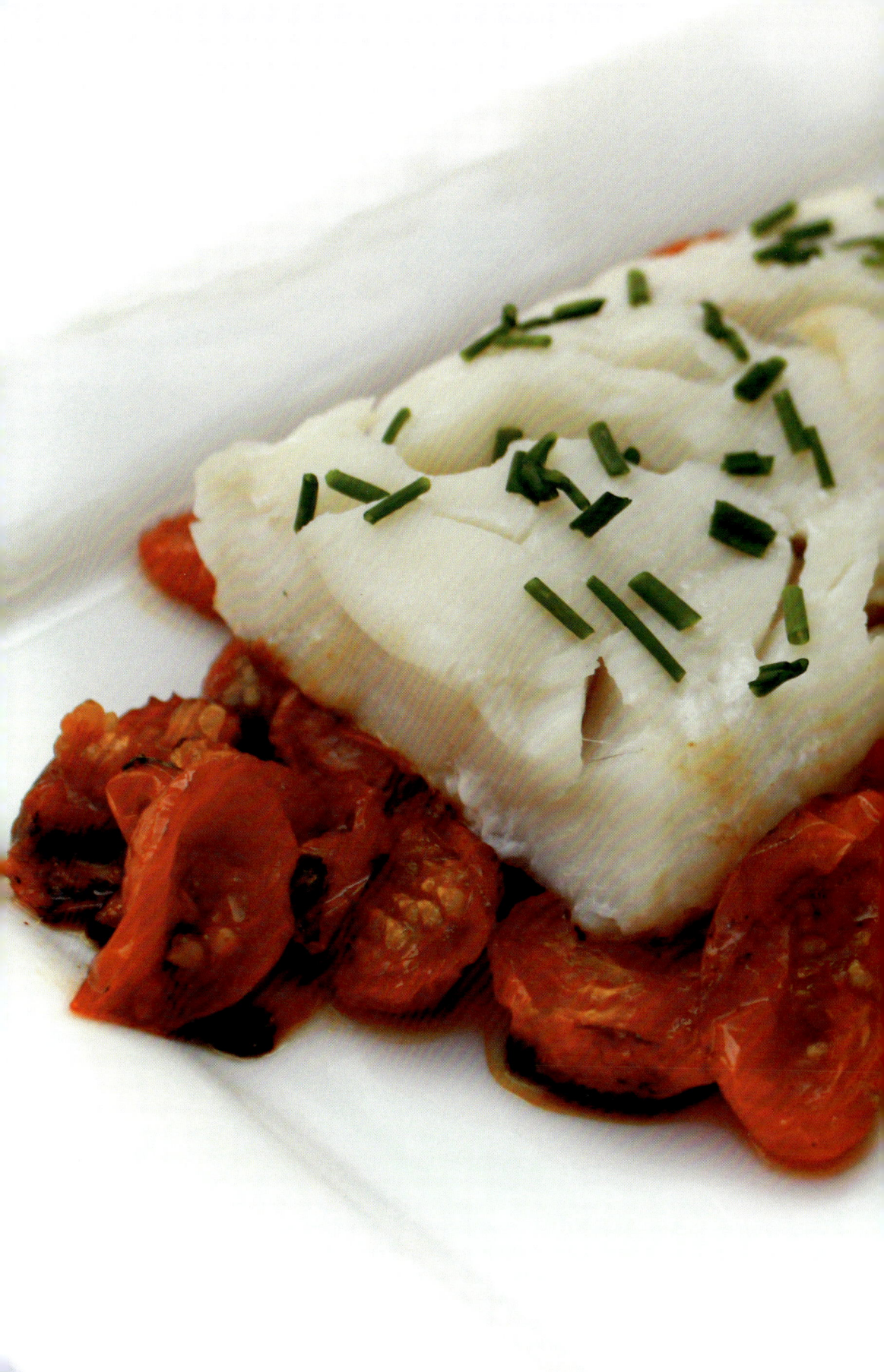

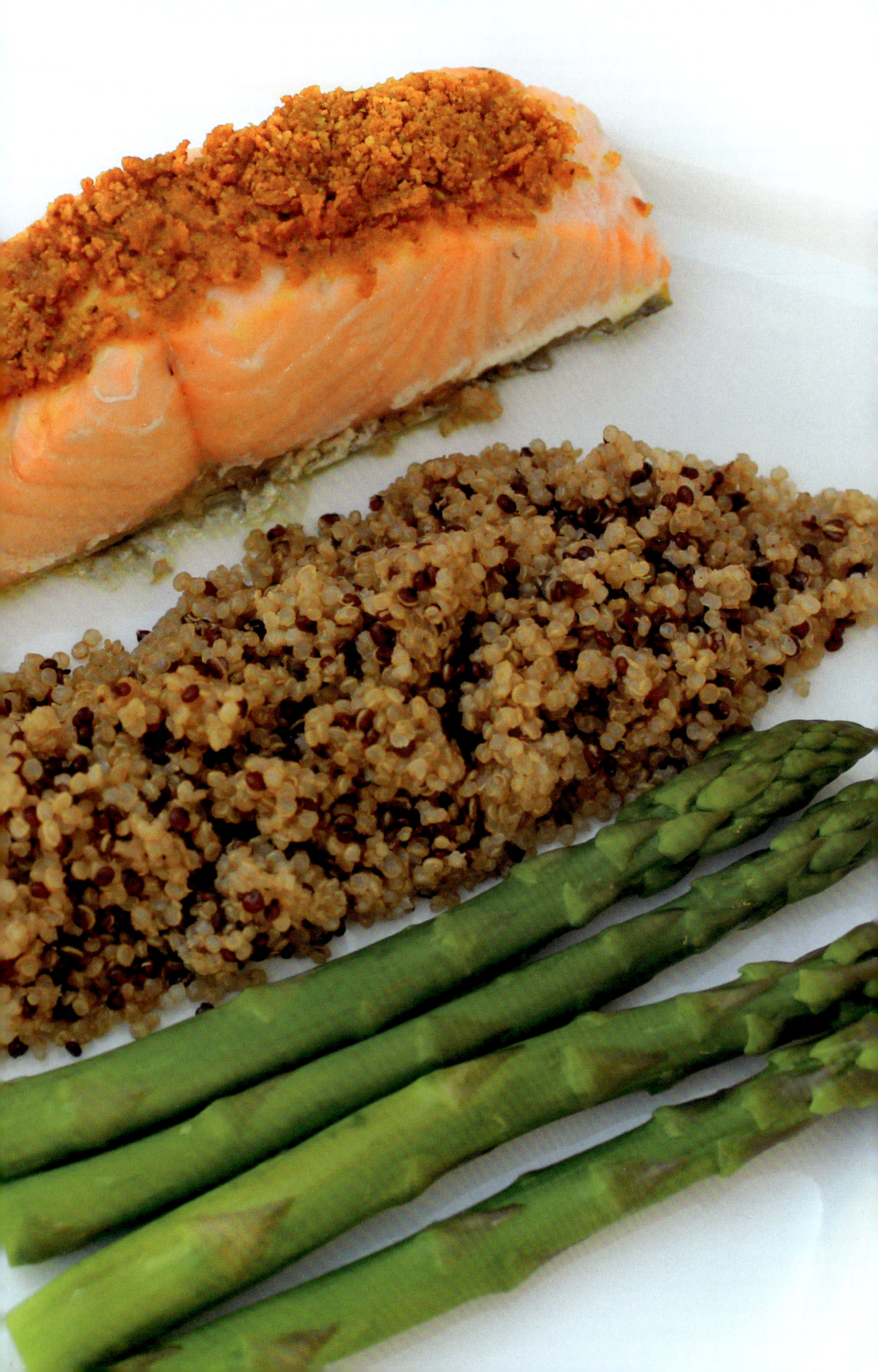

BAKED SALMON WITH QUINOA

INGREDIENTS

Ground almonds
Turmeric
Sundried tomatoes
1 piece of salmon
Asparagus
1 serving of pre-cooked quinoa

INSTRUCTIONS

Preheat oven to 180° C.

Mix together the ground almonds, turmeric and sundried tomatoes until you have a nice paste. Carefully spoon this over the salmon. Place the salmon on a baking tray and cook in the preheated oven for around 12 minutes.

Bring a pot of water to a boil and cook the asparagus for about 4 minutes.

Once cooked, plate salmon on a bed of quinoa and top of asparagus.

NOTE

THE PRE-COOKED QUINOA CAN BE SERVED COLD OR YOU CAN ZAP IT IN THE MICROWAVE UNTIL IT IS WARM.

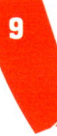

BEEF STIR-FRY

INGREDIENTS

- Sirloin steak
- 2 tbsp. of Sesame oil
- Stir-fry vegetables
- 1 small red chilli, diced
- 5cm piece of root ginger, thinly sliced
- 1 Garlic clove, thinly sliced
- A handful of peanuts, roughly chopped

INSTRUCTIONS

Trim steak, oil, season and pan-fry the steak to your liking.

Heat a wok or frying pan to a high heat with the sesame oil. Add your garlic ginger chilli and vegetables and fry for just a few minutes.

Remove vegetables from the wok and place on a plate. Slice the steak, and layer over the vegetables.

Sprinkle with chilli and peanuts to dress.

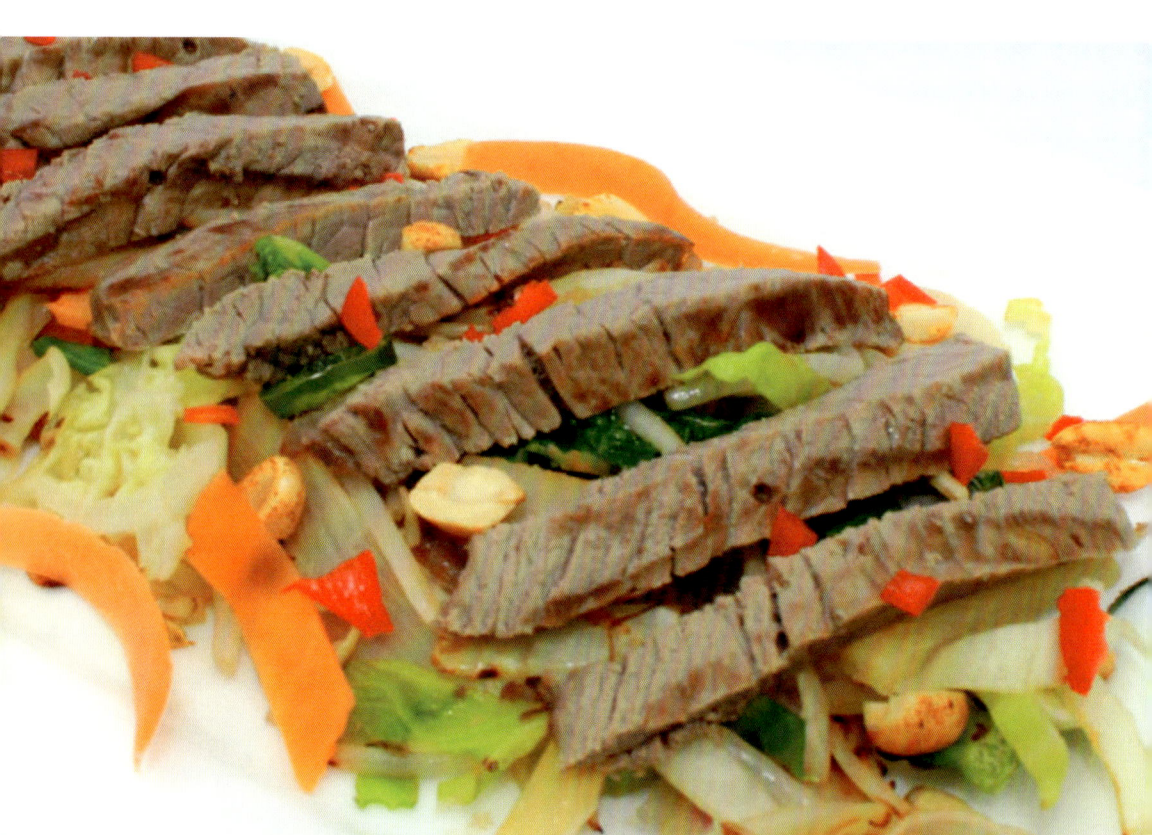

LEMON CHICKEN

INGREDIENTS

Juice and zest of two lemons.

2 tbsp. of Olive oil

1 small chicken breast

A handful of rocket leaves

A small piece of Feta cheese, crumbled

INSTRUCTIONS

Preheat the oven to 180° C. Squeeze the juice of the lemons and Olive oil into a dish and add the chicken. Leave to marinate for 20 minutes or longer.

Bake for about 15-20 minutes.

Place the chicken on the plate with the rocket and feta and dress with the lemon zest.

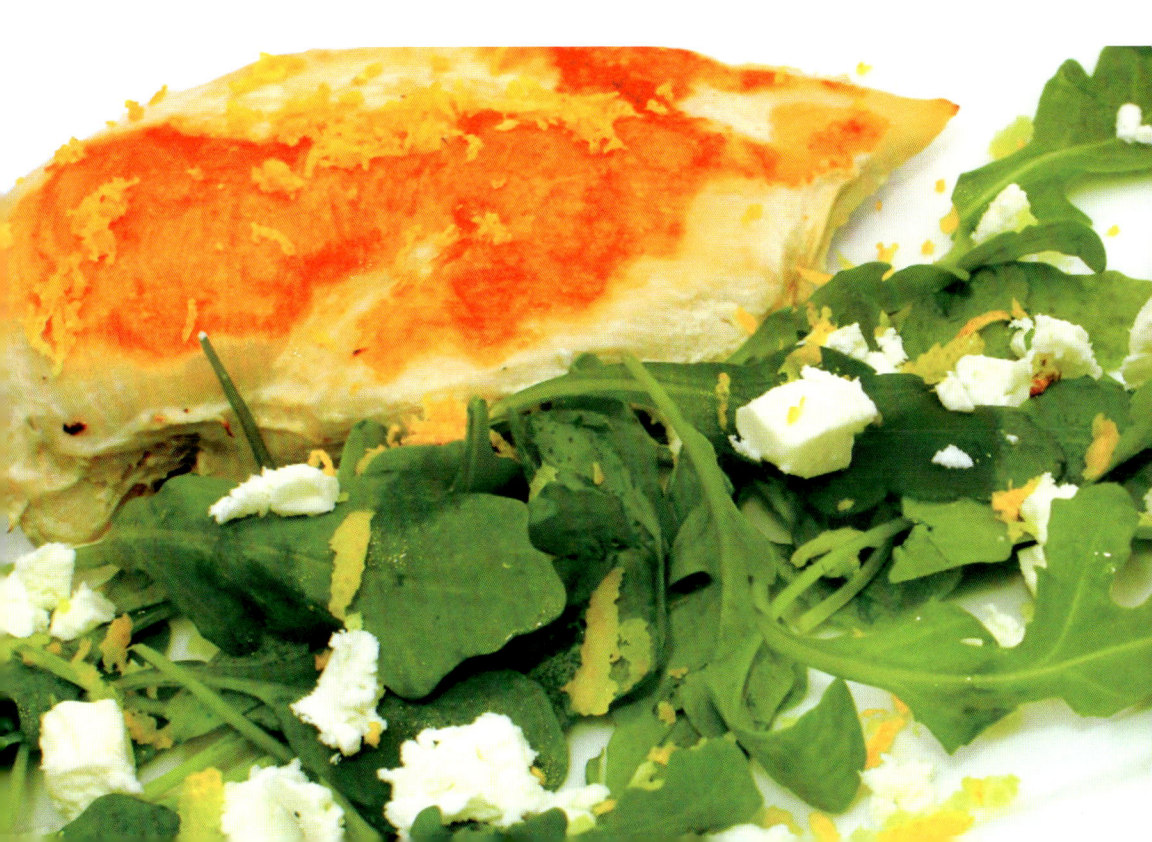

CHICKEN WITH RICE NOODLES

INGREDIENTS

Rice noodles

Red chilli, minced

Spring onion, minced

Sugar snap peas

A few pieces of pre-cooked chicken, shredded

Coriander

INSTRUCTIONS

Bring a pot of water to a boil. Turn off the heat and add the rice noodles, making sure they are completely submerged. Every minute or two, give the noodles a stir to loosen them up; this could take up to 10 minutes.

Once the noodles are cooked, drain and place in a pasta bowl. Mix in the chicken, red chili, spring onion, and sugar snap peas.

Garnish with a few coriander leaves.

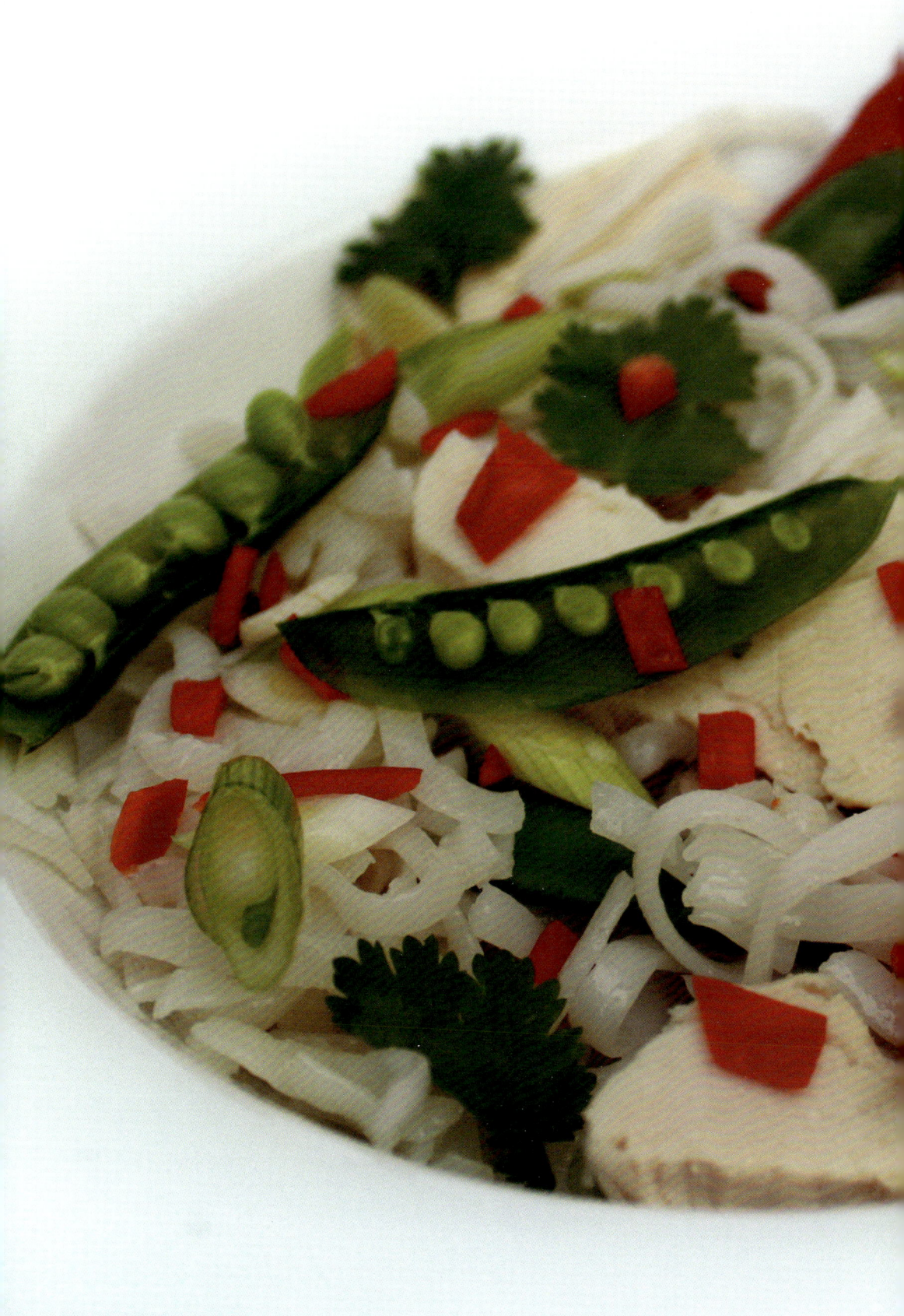

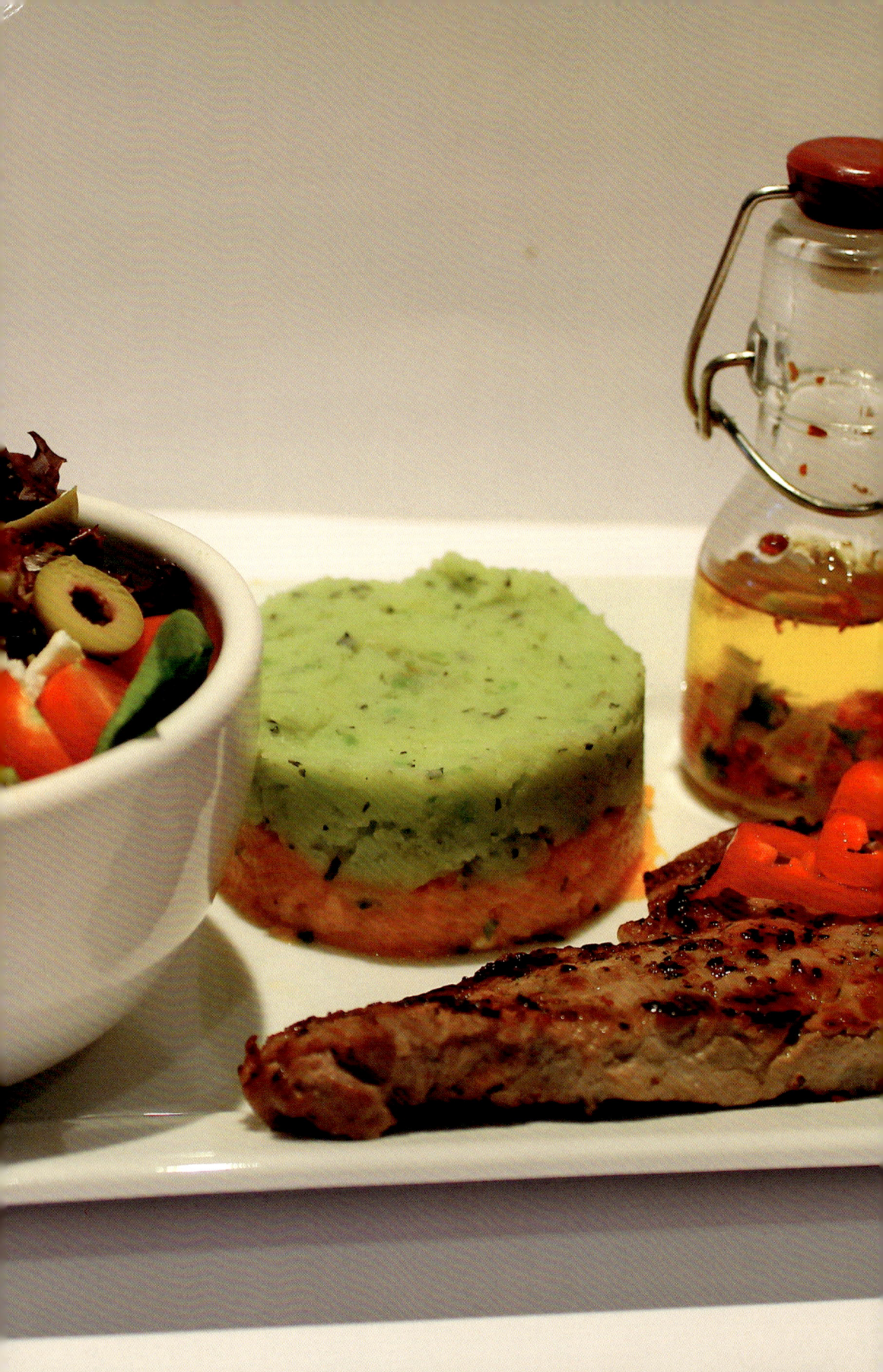

STEAK WITH TWIN MASH

INGREDIENTS

1 potato, peeled and chopped

1 sweet potato, peeled and chopped

A handful of peas

1 piece of sirloin steak

Salt and pepper to taste

2 small knobs of butter

Coriander, chopped

INSTRUCTIONS

Place the chopped potato and sweet potato in a saucepan of water and bring to a boil. Cook until they become soft and ready to mash.

While the potatoes are cooking, boil a small pan of water and cook the peas.

Season the steak with a little salt and pepper. Heat a griddle pan on high heat and cook your steak to your own liking. Once cooked, cover in foil and set aside.

Mash the sweet potato with a small knob of butter and a small handful of chopped coriander. Mash the white potato with a small knob of butter and the peas until you have a nice green texture.

Spoon the mash into a cake ring to give you the perfect stack. Place the steak on your plate with the mash and serve with a green salad.

10 LIGHT BITES

Light bites are a great alternative to processed snacks. These are full of protein, making them a healthy choice and also a great pre- or post-workout snack.

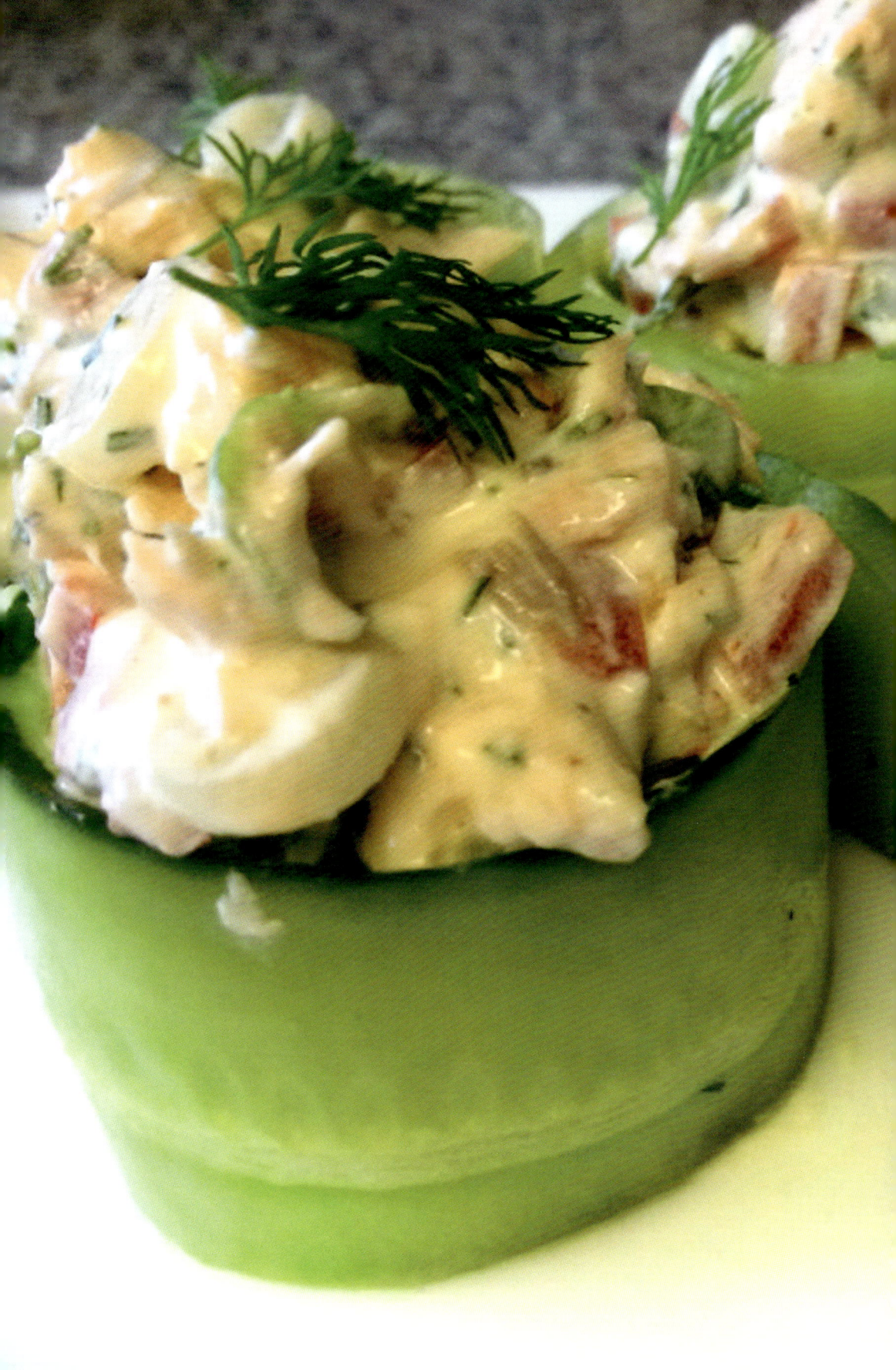

DOUBLE STACK PROTEIN

INGREDIENTS

Half of an avocado

A small tin of tuna

1 red bell pepper, diced

Sesame seeds

Salt and pepper to taste

INSTRUCTIONS

Fill the halved avocado with the tuna and a few small pieces of red pepper. Dress with the sesame seeds and season to taste.

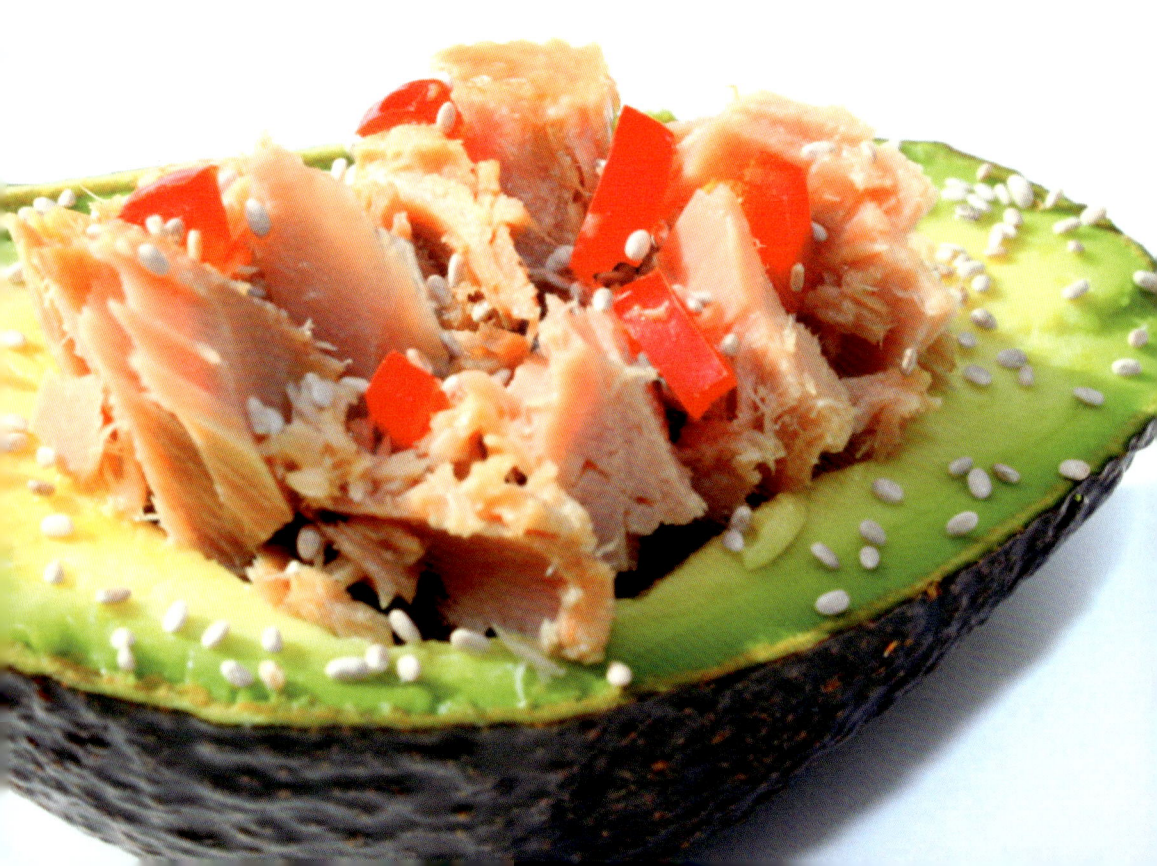

POWER FRIES AND PROTEIN DIP

INGREDIENTS

1 sweet potato, peeled and sliced into small wedges

Chili oil

Paprika

1 avocado, peeled and mashed

Juice from half of a lime

INSTRUCTIONS

Preheat the oven to 220° C. Place the sweet potato wedges into a plastic bag with some oil and paprika, and shake to coat all over.

Spread the wedges on a baking tray and cook for about 20 minutes, turning occasionally.

Combine the mashed avocado with the lime juice.

When the wedges are nicely browned and crispy, serve on a plate with the avocado-lime dip.

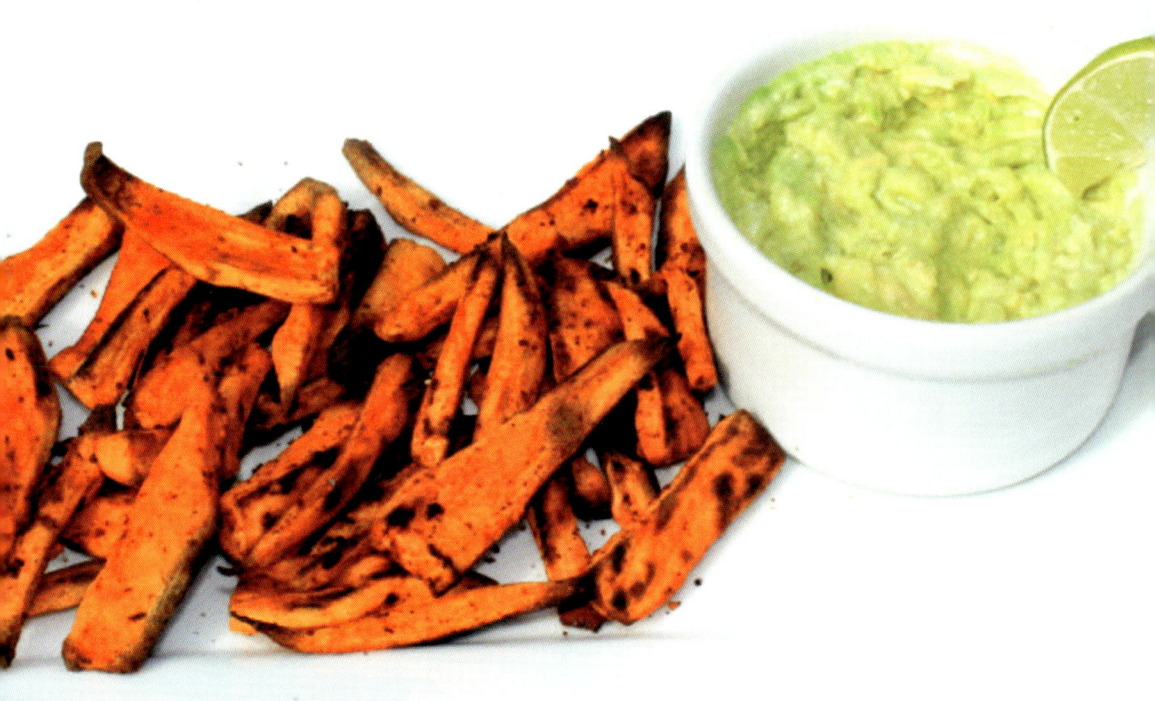

ZUCCHINI PIZZA BITES

INGREDIENTS

Zucchini, sliced

Tomato purée

Mozzarella

Mixed Italian herbs

INSTRUCTIONS

Preheat oven to 180° C.

Spread tomato purée on each slice of zucchini. Add a small piece of mozzarella and a sprinkle of Italian seasoning.

Bake in a preheated oven for 8 minutes.

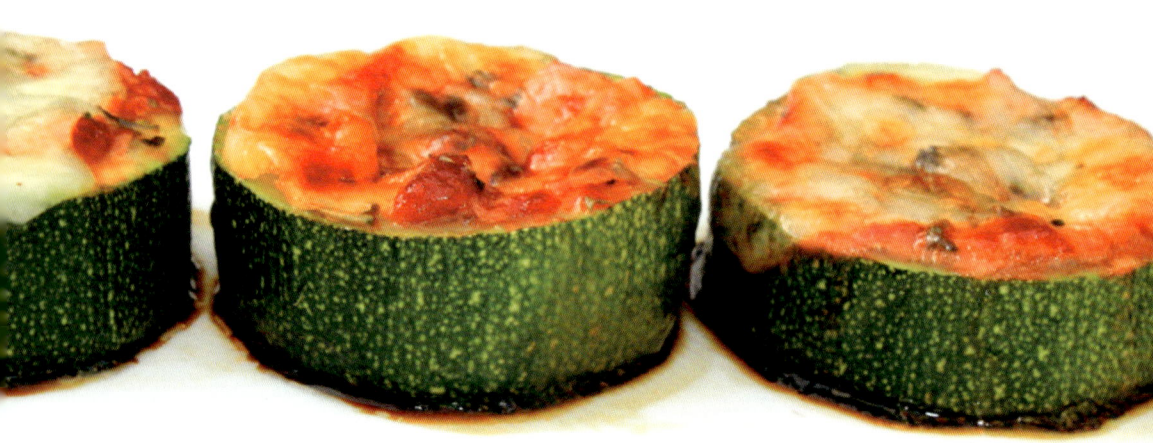

CALAMARI AND BEAN SALAD

INGREDIENTS

10 calamari rings, sliced into rings about 8mm

A generous dash of chilli flakes.

Olive oil

100ml of butter beans

Rocket leaves

1 small red chilli, sliced

Juice from a lime

INSTRUCTIONS

Gently fry your calamari rings with a drizzle of Olive oil and a good dash of chilli flakes for 3 to 4 minutes, turning halfway through. When cooked, remove from pan and set aside to cool.

Mix the cooled calamari, rocket and butter beans together. Dress with a few thin slices of red chilli and a good squeeze of lime.

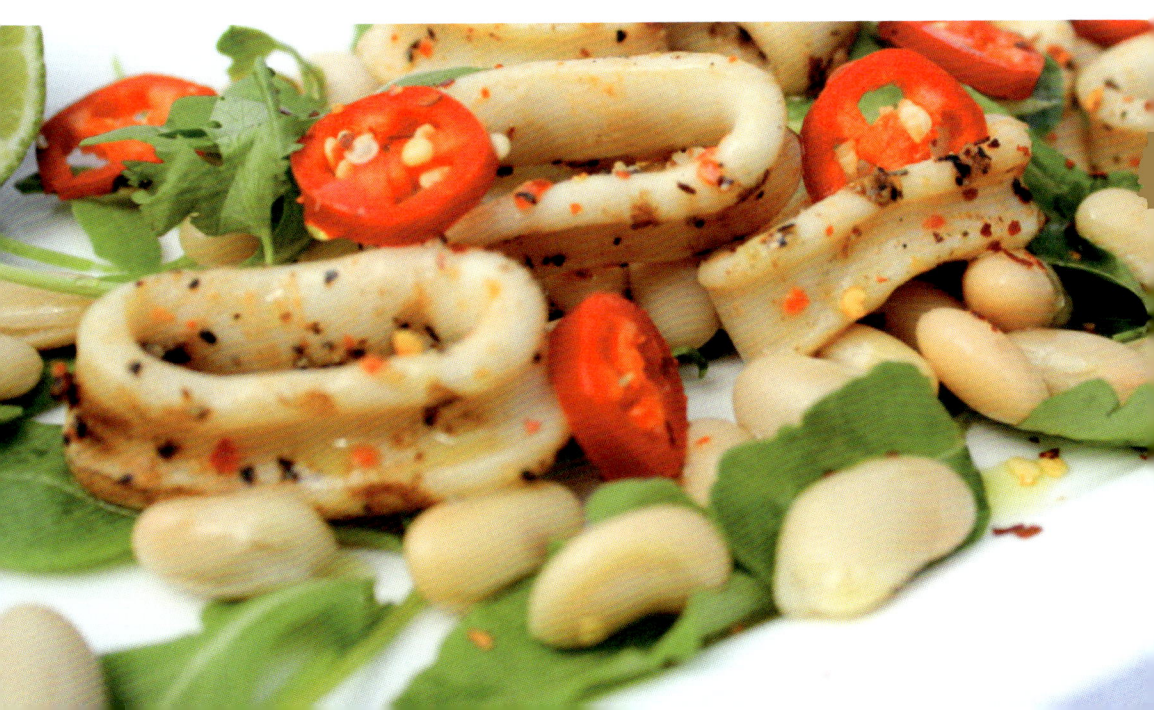

MIXED GREENS

INGREDIENTS

- Asparagus
- Mange tout
- Walnuts
- Walnut oil

INSTRUCTIONS

Bring a pot of water to a boil, add the asparagus and cook for 3 minutes.

Bring another pot of water to a boil and cook the mange tout for 1.5 minutes.

Serve both with a sprinkle of walnuts and a drizzle of walnut oil.

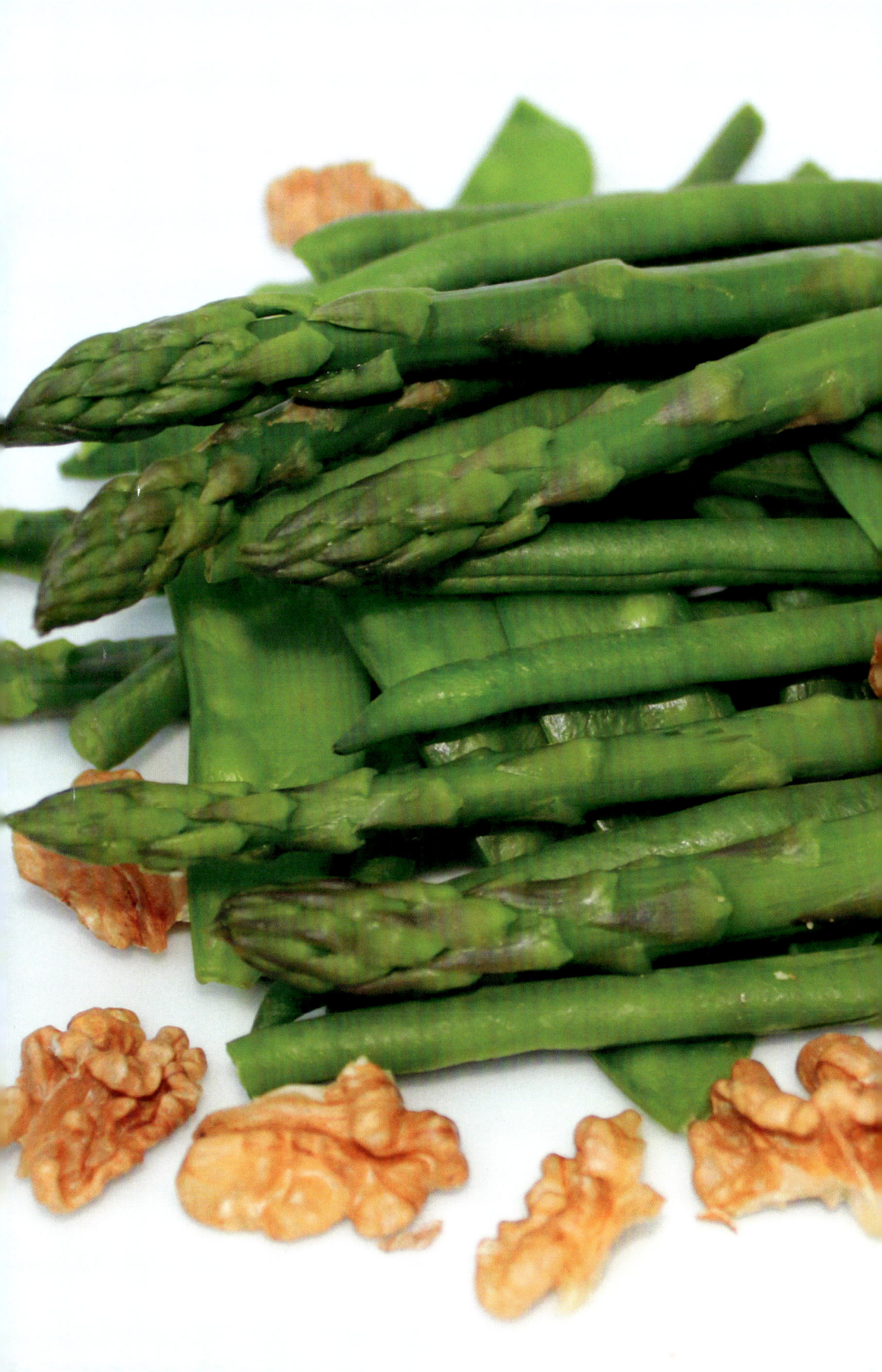

GRILLED PEACHES

INGREDIENTS

- Coconut oil
- 1 peach, sliced in half
- Greek yoghurt
- Crushed hazelnuts
- Honey

INSTRUCTIONS

Heat the coconut oil in a grill pan. Place the peaches skin side up, and cook for about 4 minutes.

Carefully remove, and top with a spoonful of Greek yoghurt. Sprinkle with crushed hazelnuts and drizzle with honey.

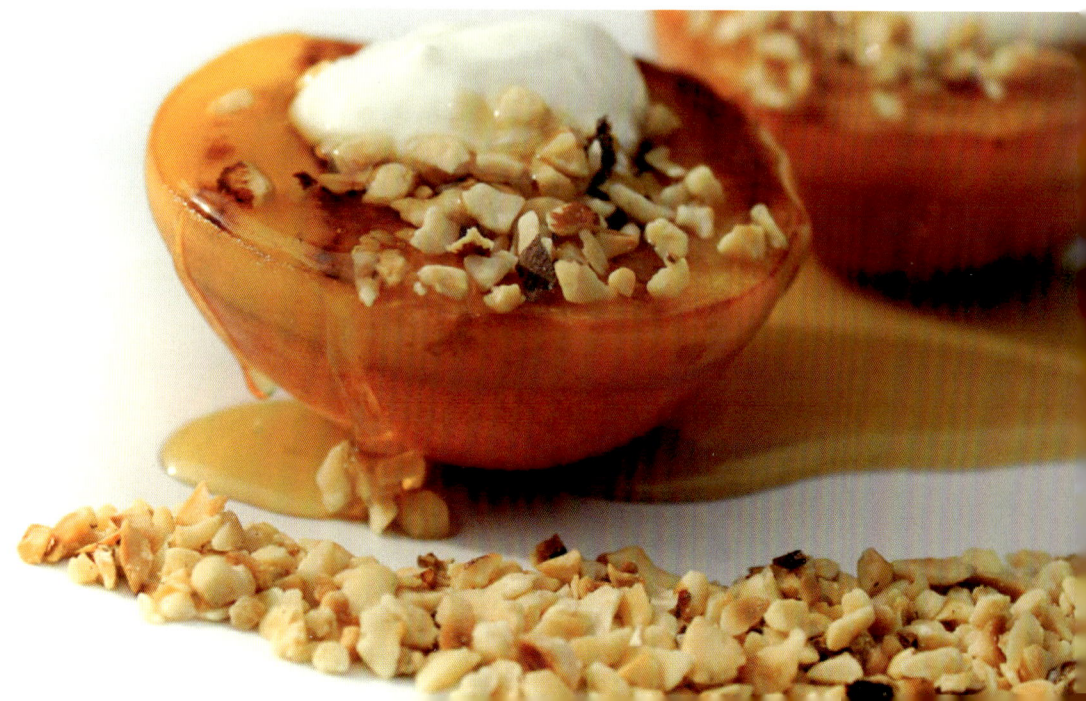

BLISS BALLS

INGREDIENTS

A handful of dates, mashed

Generous spoonful of peanut butter

2 tsp. cocoa powder

A few drops of vanilla extract

Crushed hazelnuts

Topping (for example, dried coconut, ground almonds, dark cocoa powder or dried raspberries)

INSTRUCTIONS

Mix together the mashed dates and the peanut butter. Add two teaspoons of cocoa powder and the vanilla extract. Mix well.

Using a tablespoon as a rough measure, form the mixture into balls and roll in a topping of your choice for the perfect snack.

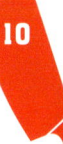

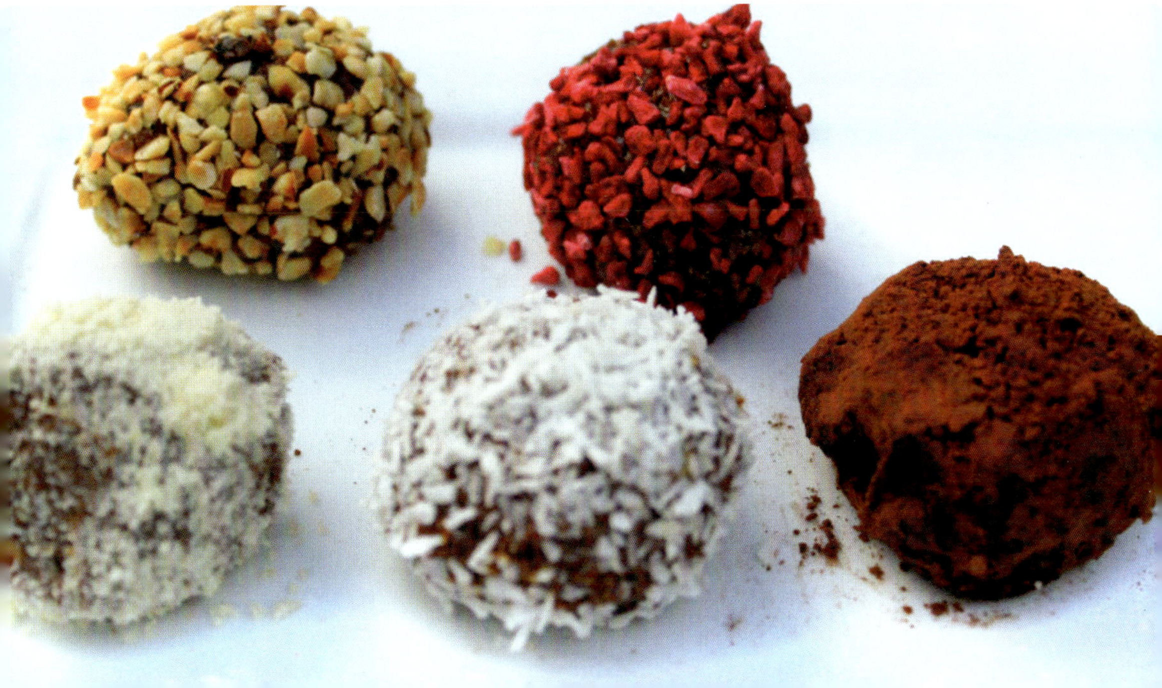

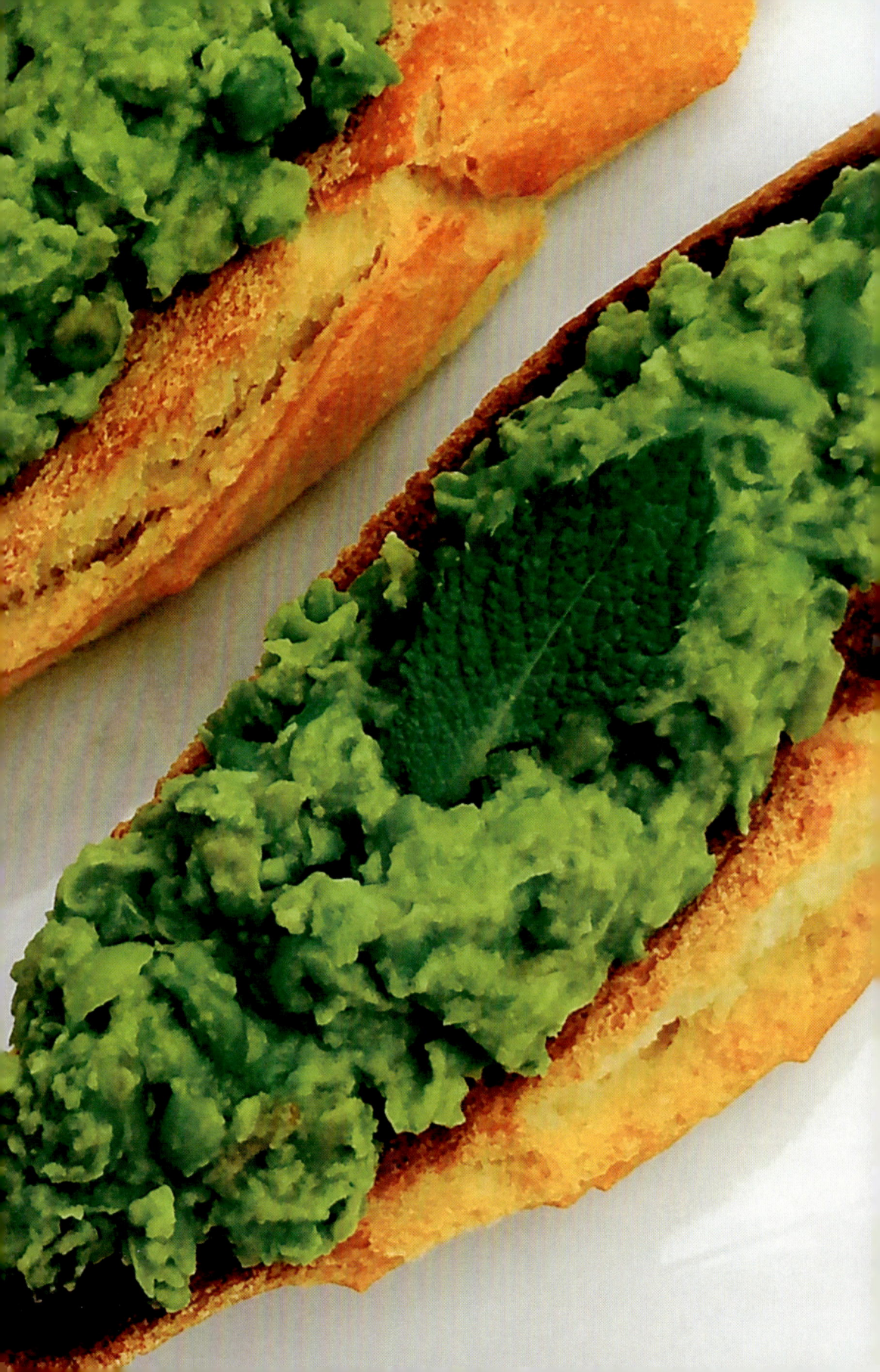

MINTED PEAS

INGREDIENTS

200g of frozen peas

8 mint leaves

2 tbsp. of Greek yoghurt

2 slices of French bread, toasted

INSTRUCTIONS

Bring a pot of water to a boil. Add the peas and cook for about 5 minutes until soft.

Drain the peas and place in a small blender. Add the mint leaves and yoghurt and give it a quick blitz.

Carefully place over your toasted bread.

LIGHT SNACK

INGREDIENTS

- 2 rice cakes
- Cottage cheese
- Cucumber, sliced
- Tomato, sliced

INSTRUCTIONS

Spread each rice cake with a generous helping of cottage cheese. Top one with cucumber and the other with tomato.

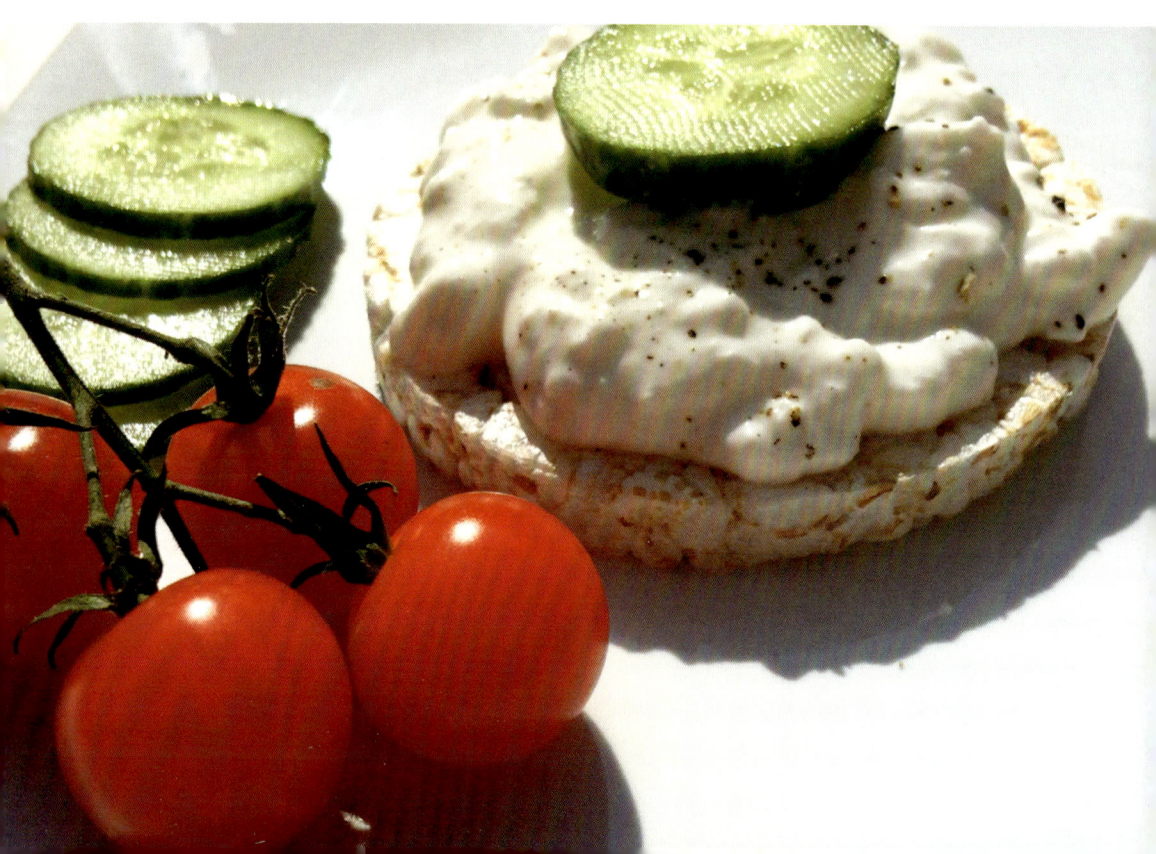

Light Bites

OPEN-FACED AVOCADO SANDWICH

INGREDIENTS

1 slice of wholemeal bread, toasted

Half of an avocado, sliced

Cherry tomatoes, halved

Rocket leaves

Parmesan cheese

INSTRUCTIONS

Top the toasted bread with the rocket, avocado, and cherry tomatoes. Top with crumbled parmesan cheese.

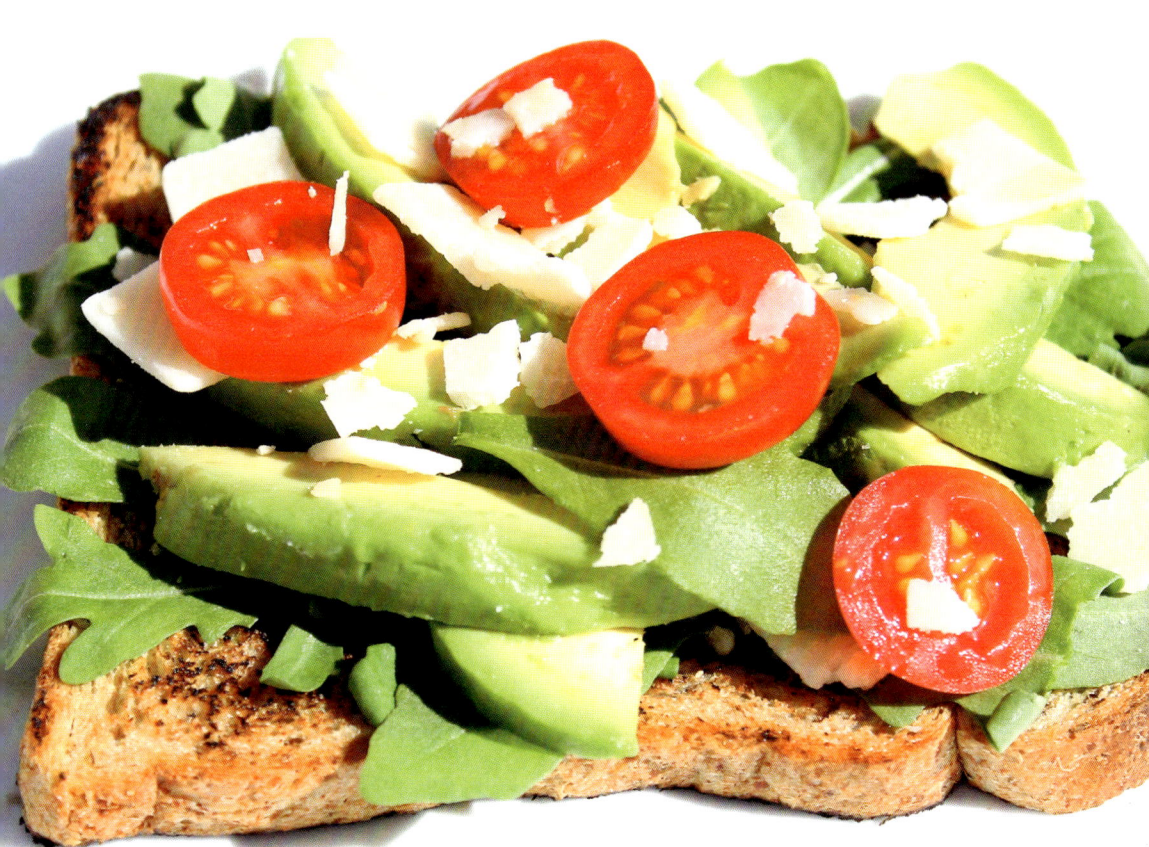

SWEET POTATO CRISPS

INGREDIENTS

1 sweet potato

Chilli oil

Paprika

Natural yoghurt

Coriander

INSTRUCTIONS

Preheat oven to 200° C.

Using a mandolin, carefully slice the sweet potato into crisp-sized bites.

In a large freezer bag, add some chilli oil and paprika. Put the sweet potato in the bag and gently shake to make sure you cover all of the potatoes.

Spread the seasoned potatoes on an oven tray and bake for 25 minutes, making sure you turn them as you go.

When they are nice and brown, remove from the oven and serve with a dip made of natural yogurt and coriander

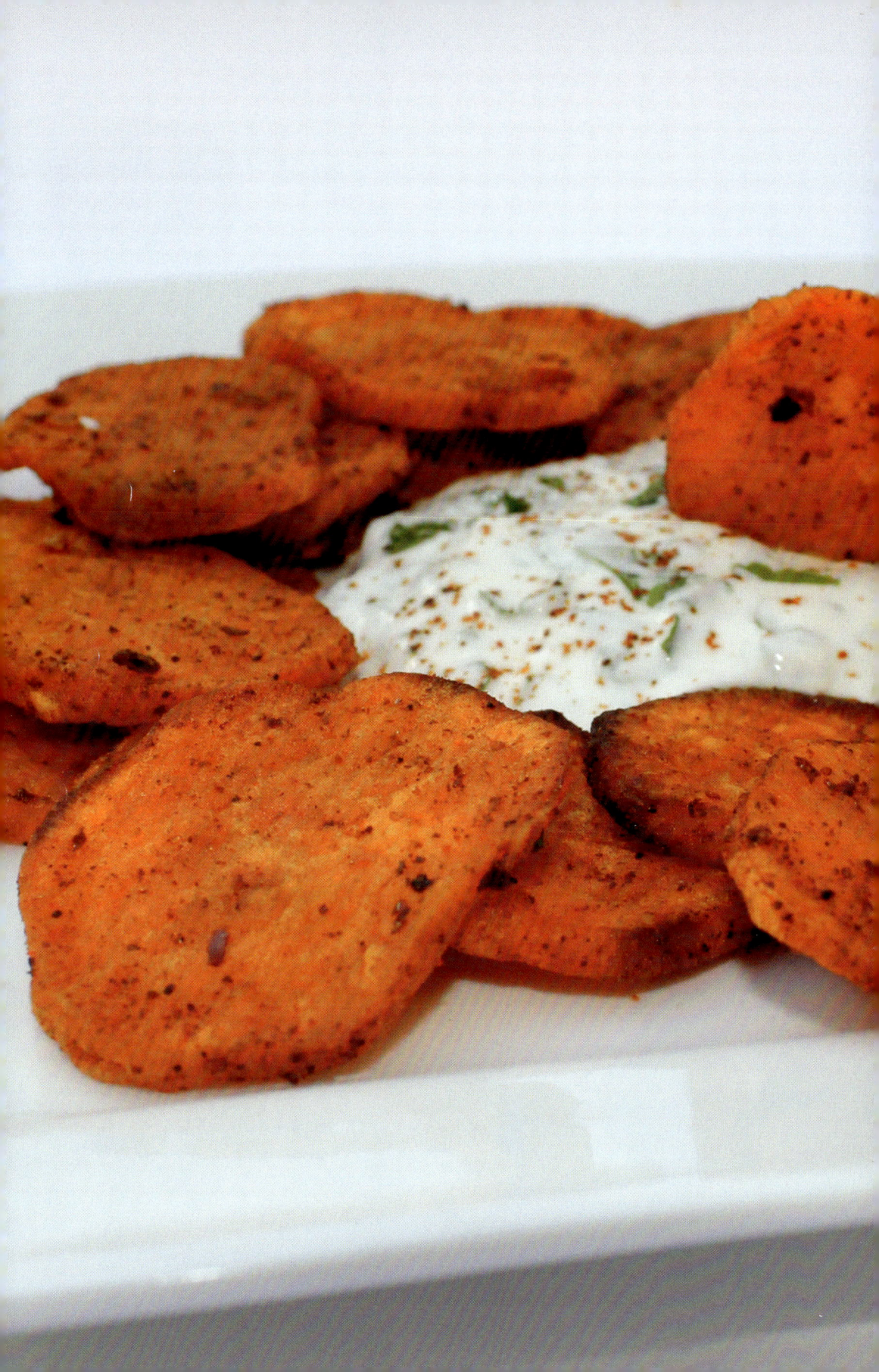

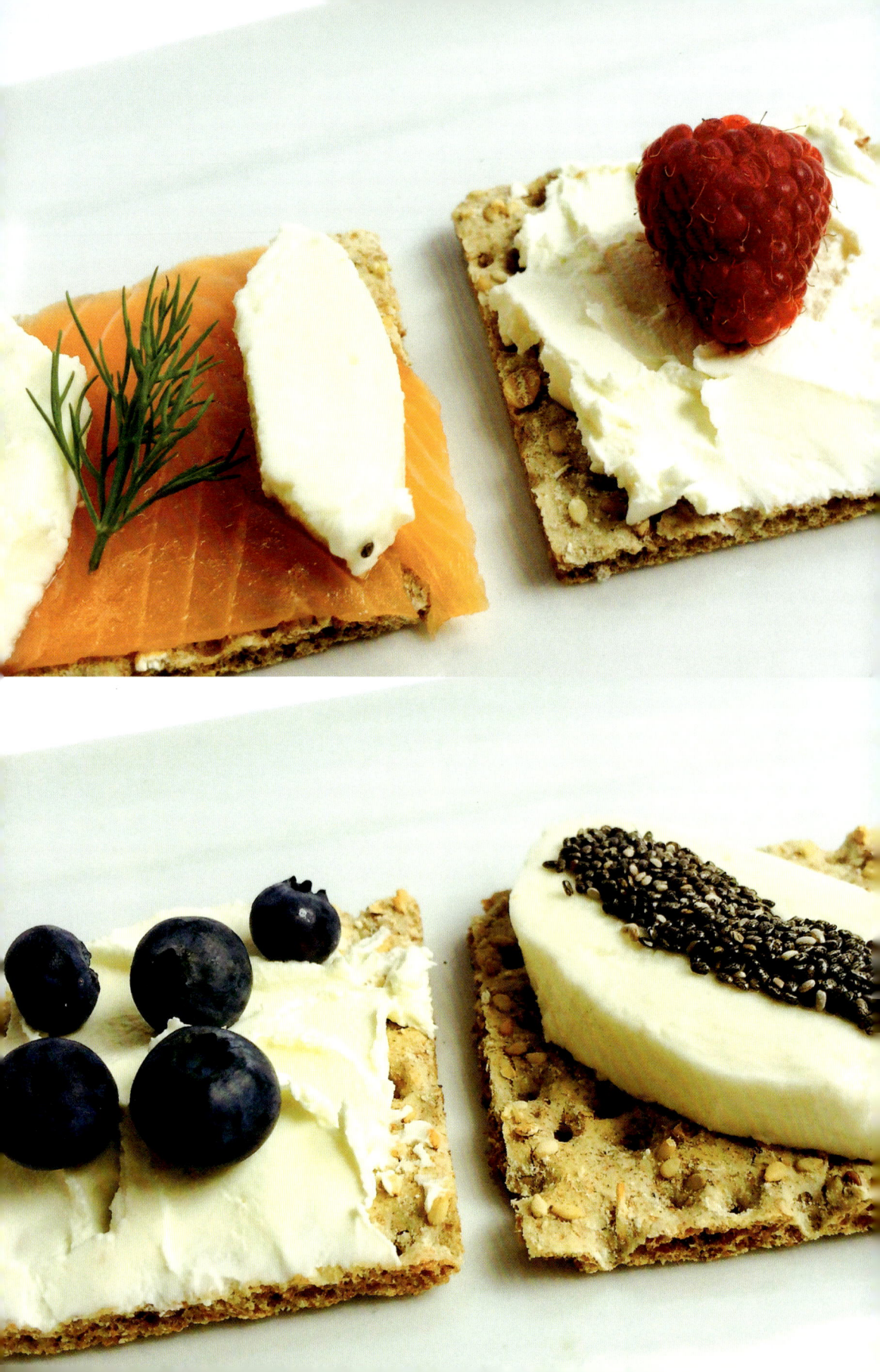

HUNGER FILLERS

INGREDIENTS

2 pieces of crispbread

Smoked salmon

Cream cheese

Mozzarella cheese

Raspberries

Blueberries

Chia seeds

INSTRUCTIONS

Spread the crispbread pieces with a thick layer of cream cheese. Top one with raspberries and blueberries and the other with smoked salmon and mozzarella. Sprinkle with chia seeds.

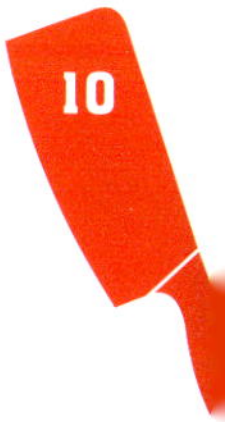

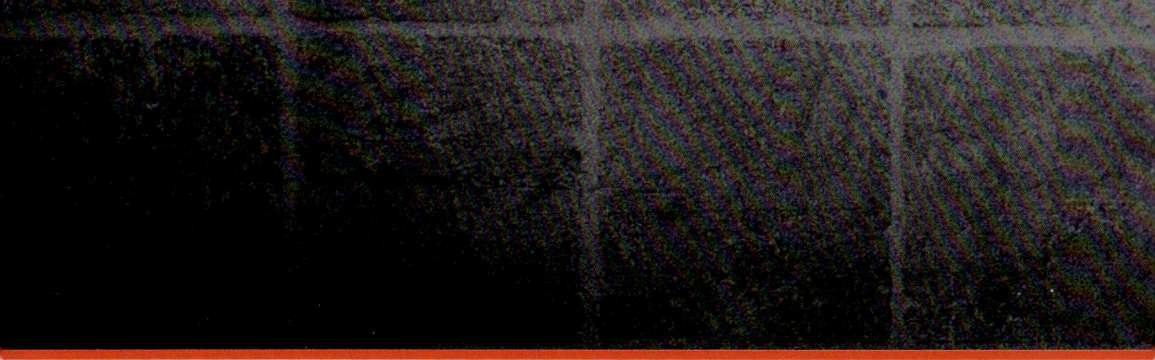

11 SMOOTHIES

Smoothies are a great way to quickly boost your energy, improve your brainpower, and get a quick powerful punch of vitamins and minerals. My smoothies include the entire daily allowance of multivitamins in a glass.

If you have a diet rich in a wide variety of vegetables and fruits, you don't need to buy expensive supplements; that's why in Men's Fit Kitchen I decided to get down and dirty with some veggies and fruits, and knock up six muscle-building smoothies for you.

There is no wrong or right way to make a smoothie; just grab your veggies and fruit and create your own mix. However, you do need to follow a rule of never having more than 3 pieces of fruit in a smoothie, as this makes the sugar content too high.

Here are six smoothies that will nourish and keep you fuelled. Just use a small piece of every ingredient and experiment in your blender. Enjoy!

GREEN MONSTER

INGREDIENTS

- Handful of spinach
- Celery
- Cucumber
- Apple
- A small piece of ginger
- Half of an avocado
- Coconut water
- Goji berries
- Chia seeds

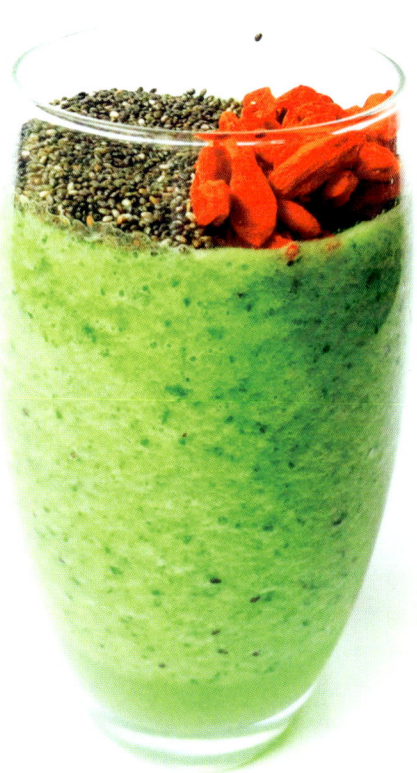

CARDIO CRUSH

INGREDIENTS

Beetroot

Mint

Ginger

Cherries

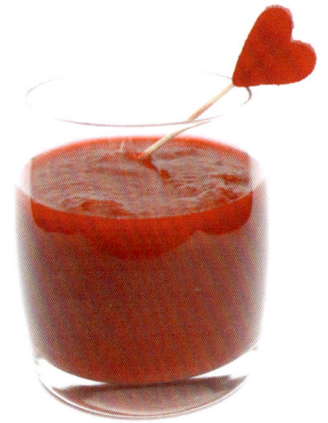

IMMUNE BOOSTER SHOT

INGREDIENTS

Pear

Ginger

Cinnamon

Tangerine

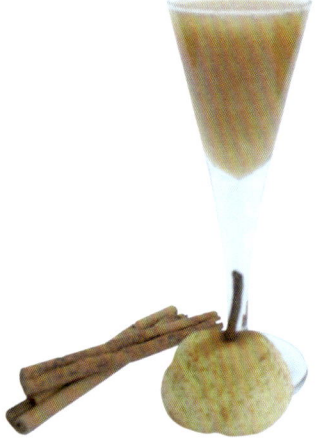

BETA BLASTER

INGREDIENTS

Carrot

Orange

Ginger

Pineapple

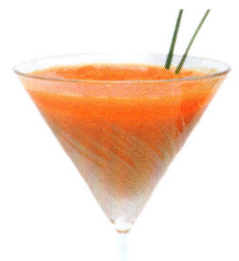
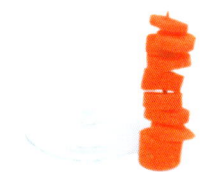

LEAN AND GREEN SHOT

INGREDIENTS

Cucumber

Kale

Spinach

Lime

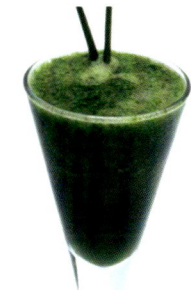

CHILLI SHOT

INGREDIENTS

Beetroot

Apple

Chilli

Red currants

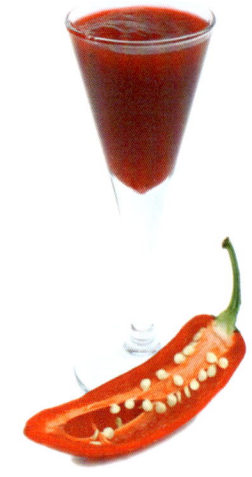

BERRY BOOSTER

INGREDIENTS

6 large strawberries

A handful of raspberries

Coconut yoghurt

Semi-skimmed milk

Hazelnuts, crushed

Honey

INSTRUCTIONS

Place strawberries, raspberries, yoghurt, honey and milk in your blender. Blitz.

Sprinkle crushed hazelnuts to finish.

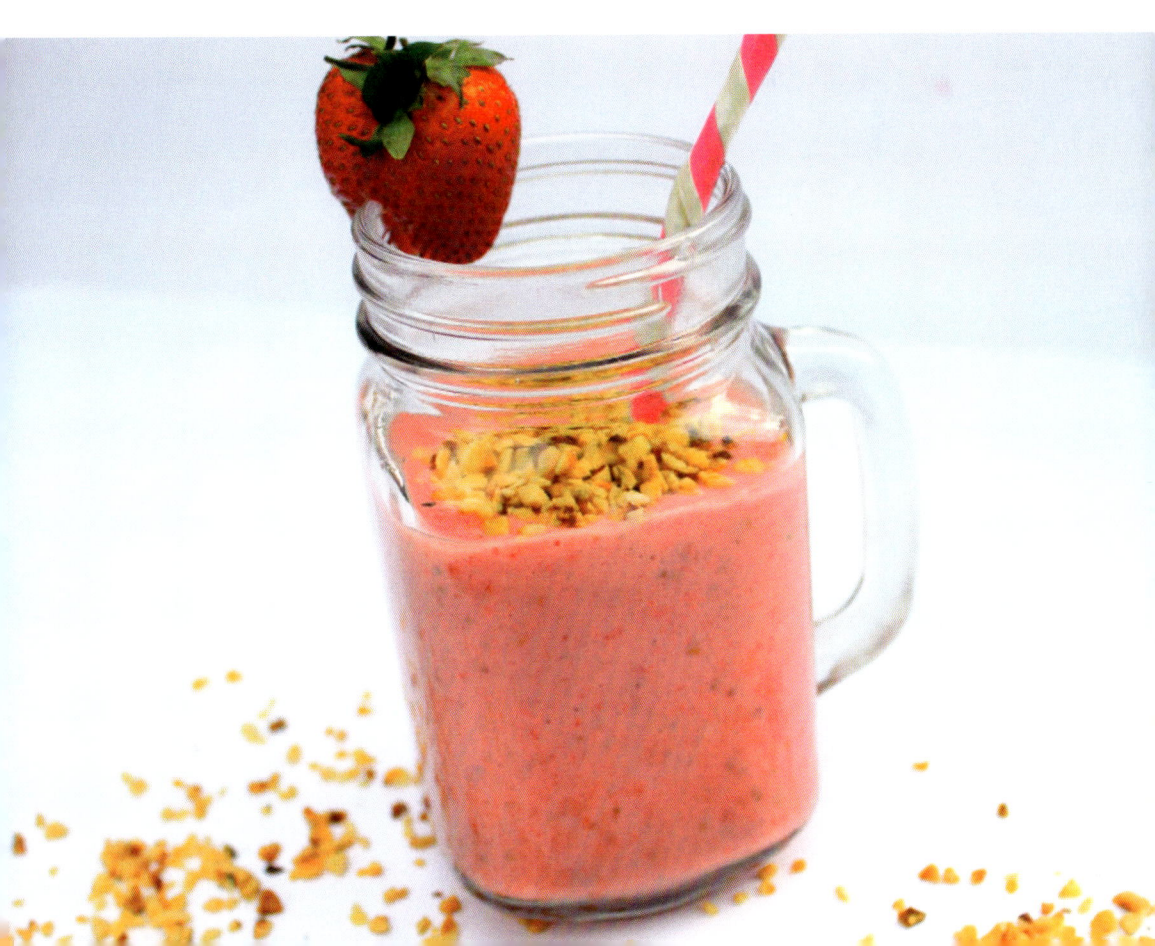

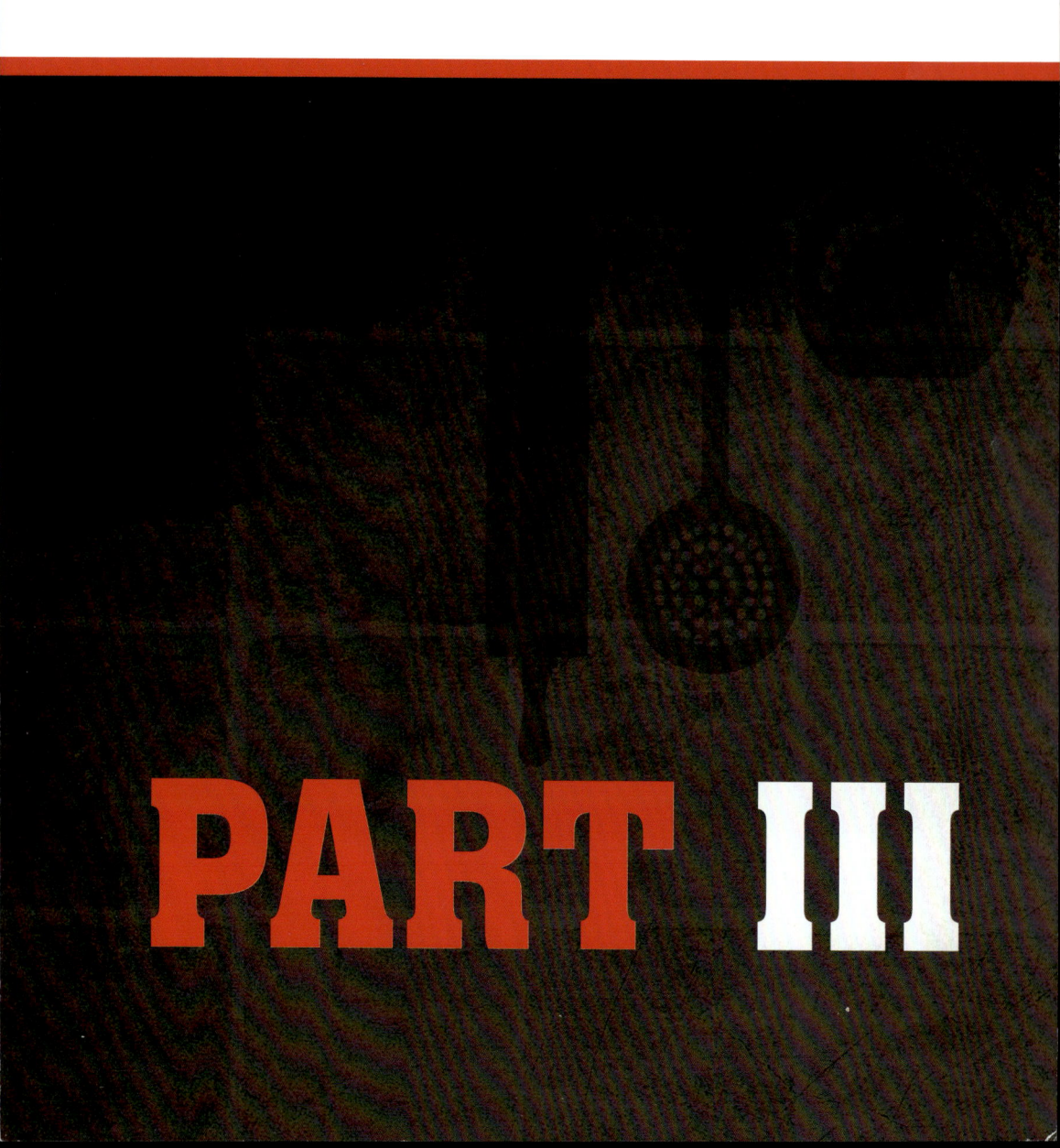

PART III

FITNESS

12 RUNNING AND GETTING STARTED

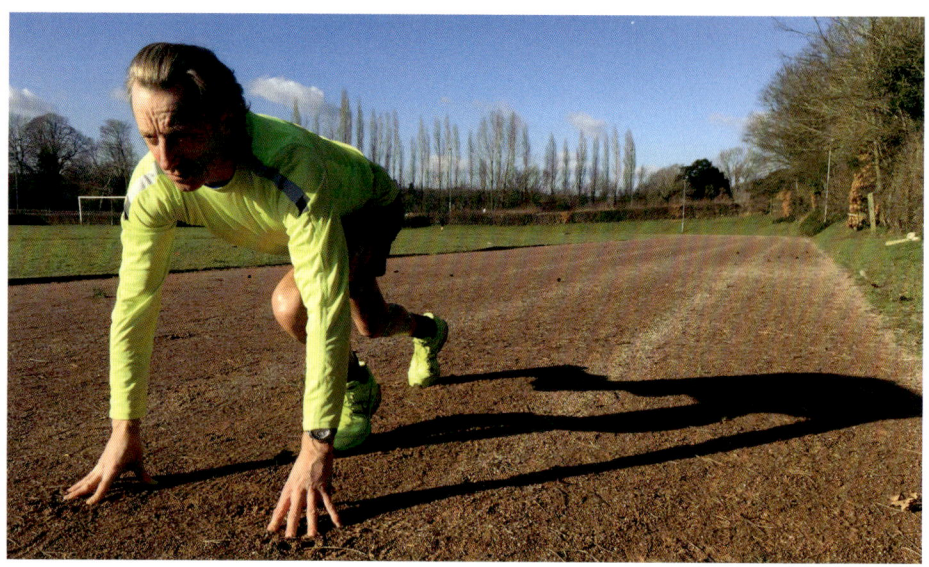

MAKING RUNNING EASY

If you are a non-runner, then this is going to be your start to the new you. The following pages will take you on a journey from a being a complete non-runner to becoming a good intermediate runner. I will show you many different skills and techniques to improve your stamina and speed with some great indoor and unique outdoor exercises to improve your overall body strength. I will also show you the benefits of hill running and why, in my opinion, this is one of the greatest ways to improve your overall strength and speed.

If you plan to lose weight and improve your running, then this book will guide you in a simple manner. Eating healthy is a great start and will help you lose weight, make you feel so much better and give you greater confidence. However, to get your desired results you must plan to train at least three times a week to start with, and the best way to get going is by walking.

WHAT YOU NEED TO GET STARTED

There are many ways to start. First, and most importantly, you need to invest in a good pair of running shoes. Running shoes vary in price from reasonably cheap to damn expensive. Don't be fooled into thinking that expensive is always the best. The best shoe for you is the one that fits you best. Put fashion aside and think comfort as these shoes are going to carry you for many miles to come.

The most important aspect of a good running shoe is that it has good cushioning in the heel to absorb most of the impact. Good shock absorption is important as your foot absorbs up to four times of your own body weight with each step you take. Therefore the best advice I can give you is to purchase your shoes from a specialized running shop. The staff in these shops will be knowledgeable about their products and take care in fitting you with the right shoe for you. You should buy a shoe at least a half a size bigger than your usual footwear as your feet will expand whilst you run.

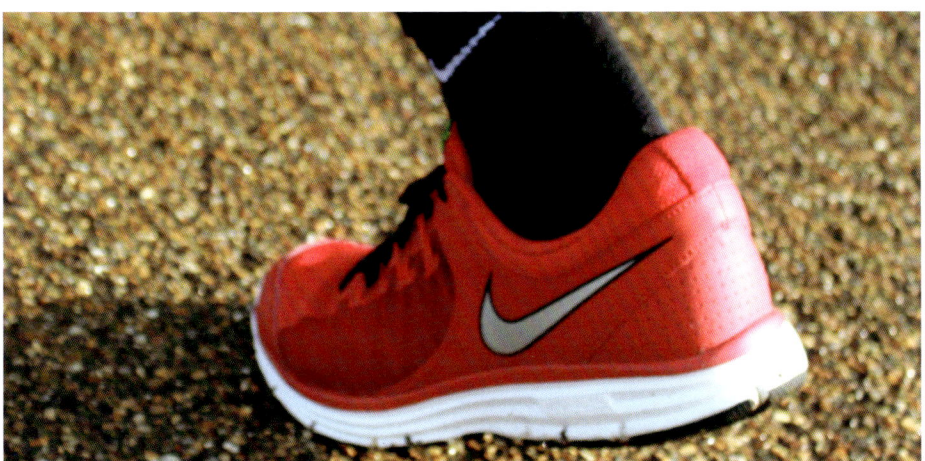

TRAINING KIT

Your next expense is going to be your training kit and you do not need to spend a fortune on this. Running clothes are designed to be comfortable and functional to make your running as easy as possible. Good quality clothing will stay dry whilst allowing moisture to pass through to the outside.

TIP

Avoid cotton at all costs! Cotton absorbs sweat and can trap in the cold and lead to chaffing and blistering. Choose shorts, tops and socks which are made of technical materials and breathable fabrics. These are designed to pull the sweat and moisture away from your skin, so in the summer they will keep you cool and in the winter they will keep the warmth in.

HATS AND GLOVES

For the winter it is paramount to keep your head and ears warm so wear a well-fitting hat that also covers your ears as you can lose as much as 40% of your body heat through your head.

Your hands also lose heat very quickly on a cold winter's day. A good pair of gloves or mitts will protect you from the elements

In the heat of the summer a baseball cap or visor will keep the sun away from your eyes. Alternatively a well-fitting pair of sunglasses is a wise investment—and don't forget to use sun cream!

WINDPROOF JACKET

It is worth investing in a good windproof jacket as wind can be one of the biggest factors to contend with on a winter's day. Look for a jacket which is breathable and waterproof, and, if you run after dark, consider a reflective one.

RUNNING TIGHTS

A lot of men like to feel the cold of the winter breeze around their legs and run in shorts. However, this doesn't keep you warm so running tights are a great way of insulating you from the cold. Running tights also have the benefit of adding a compression layer to your body which will stimulate blood flow to your legs.

BEATING THE BOREDOM

Many first-time runners look for excuses as to why they do not like running, and the one that always hits the top of the list is boredom. A great way to avoid this is to use headphones and a portable music player. However, it is important to always make sure that you can still hear noises around you for safety, so never have the volume too loud unless you are in a safe place to run.

For example, I enjoy 5K and 10K races and will load only enough music for my planned time. I also organise my playlists so that the beat will be much faster toward the end to drive me to a faster time.

The other great way to beat the boredom is to choose some appealing routes for your run. You can't beat running through the countryside or on trail runs through the forest

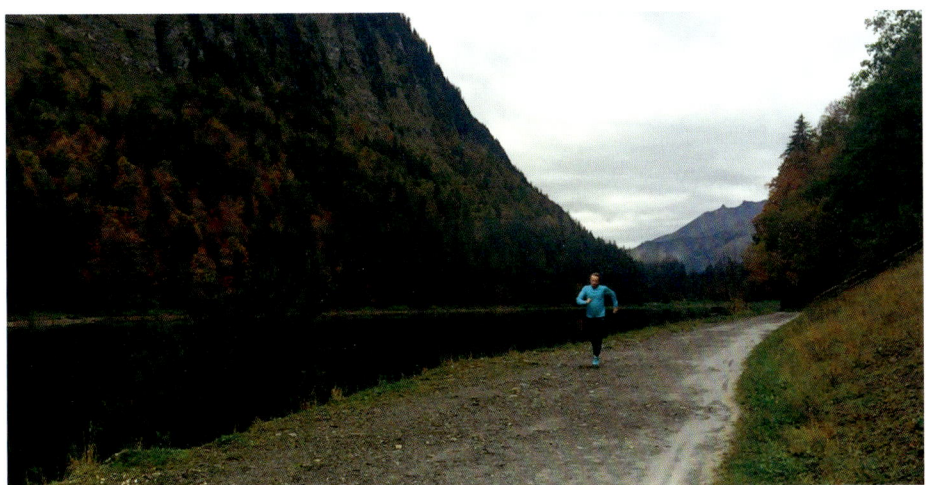

where nature is at its best. One of my favourite places to run is around Lake Montriond in Morzine, France where I have my lovely ski chalet. Being in the mountains also gives me the opportunity for some challenging trail and hill runs.

Try to get a friend, work colleague or neighbour to run with you; this way you need never get bored and you will motivate each other to improve your running skills.

A WORD OF CAUTION

If you are a non-runner, then the worst thing that you can do is lace up and try to run like Usain Bolt. The chances are that you will

- injure yourself,
- pull a muscle,
- hate it,
- want to give up, or
- even end up in hospital.

Running should be enjoyable, so it is very important that you take your time to slowly build up your distance, stamina, and strength. Most of us have heard the saying "Learn to walk before you can run," and that is exactly how we are going to start: by power walking and slowly increasing your aerobic ability to break into running. Power walking has lots of great benefits:

- It's a great introduction to running.
- It's low impact.
- It tones your body.
- It improves heart and lung function.
- It burns calories.
- It's great for the abs.
- It gives you more energy.
- It boosts circulation.

WARM UP, COOL DOWN AND STRETCH

Warming up is an absolutely vital part of exercising but sadly one that often gets ignored. Warming up not only helps you perform better but it can also help to prevent injuries. I suggest you warm up before you do any of the exercises or the running and walking workouts.

When you are heading outdoors to do your running or walking workouts, it is a good idea to spend a couple of minutes walking at a moderate pace and gradually build up the speed, so that by the end of the two minutes you are walking at a good, brisk pace. This will help increase your core body temperature, and the motion of walking is a great way of lubricating your joints and muscles so that when you start exercising fully your muscles are more pliable, making the exercise easier. Bear in mind that on a boiling hot day your body temperature will naturally be higher, as opposed to a cold day when you may want to spend longer warming up. As a good rule of thumb, always ensure you feel warm before you start exercising.

WARMING UP

Before you commence any running you need to prepare your body for the demands that you will be asking of it. Warming up is an essential part of your training program and prevents injury. Your warm-up stretches play an important role in your training as these lengthen your muscles by keeping them healthy and flexible. Stretching will also increase your heart rate and mobilise your joints.

Your muscles are more prone to injury when they are cold and tight so I start my stretching with a small power walk to warm up my body and muscles. After about 5 minutes of power walking, and only once I feel warm, I go through a series of static stretching before I run. To date, I have never had an injury!

COOLING DOWN

Many people think once they have finished running it's okay to just stop straight away. This should be avoided at all costs. You need to slowly reduce the pace and wind down, slowly bringing your body back to its pre-exercise state. This will help reduce any tightness and soreness and help with the removal of any lactic acid you have built up.

Your cool-down only takes a few minutes after a steady run and you do this by slowing your pace to a moderate walking pace. Follow this up with some more stretching to relieve any tightness. After a hard running session or after hill running, it is essential that you go through the stretching program to prevent post-workout stiffness which can last for days.

In short, always make sure you warm up, stretch, cool down, and stretch as this will prevent muscle pain and injury.

TIP

- Hold each stretch for 20-30 seconds.
- Stretch after your body is warm.
- Never over stretch.
- If it's painful, then stop.
- Don't forget your post-run stretch.

STRETCHING

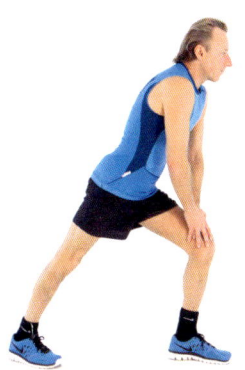

Calf stretch—Step back with one leg, keeping the heel down and both feet pointing forwards. Rest your hands on the bent leg. Hold for 20-30 seconds on each leg.

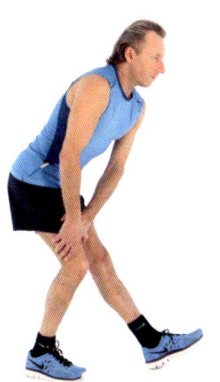

Hamstring stretch—Standing straight, bend one leg and extend the other out straight with the heel on the floor and toes pointing up. Place both hands on the bent leg and stick your bottom out to feel the stretch along the back of your straight leg. Hold for 20-30 seconds on each leg.

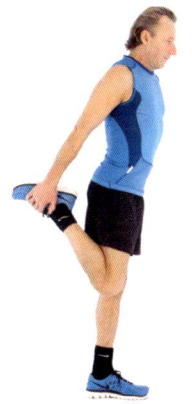

Quad stretch—Standing with good posture, bend one leg behind you and gently hold the foot or sock of the bent leg. Push your hips forward to feel the stretch in the front of your thigh. Keep the supporting knee slightly bent. Hold for 20-30 seconds on each leg.

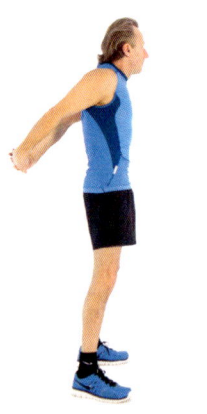

Chest stretch—Standing with good posture, take your arms behind you, and lift your shoulders up and back to feel the chest stretch. Hold for 20-30 seconds.

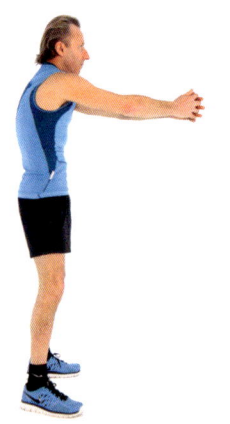

Back stretch—Stand with good posture, knees soft and tummy pulled in. Take your arms in front of you and imagine you are hugging a big beach ball. Feel the stretch in back. Hold for 20-30 seconds.

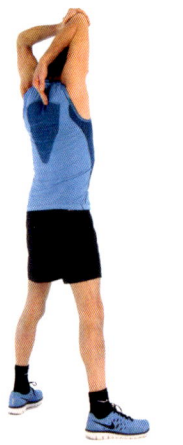

Triceps stretch—Stand with a strong, firm, straight back, knees slightly bent and tummy pulled in. Lift one arm up and bend it behind your head, aiming to get your hand between your shoulders. Hold for 20-30 seconds on each arm.

POWER WALKING

Walking is one of the simplest forms of exercise and an excellent natural way to enhance both your health and fitness. Although, generally speaking, it's a low-impact form of exercise, by altering the level of intensity via speed and incline your heart will be pumping and you will start to improve your cardio fitness straight away.

When walking you still need to dress appropriately as you may need to be ready for all kinds of weather. Here are some guidelines to follow:

- Wear layers so that you can add or remove items for temperature control.
- Wear a wind- and waterproof jacket on cooler and wetter days.
- Wear high-visibility items on darker days or if you are walking in the evenings.
- Wear a woollen hat and gloves on cold days.
- Wear a cap and sunglasses to keep the sun off your face on hot days.
- Make sure you have pockets for your phone, keys, etc., and carry a small amount of cash for emergencies.
- Carry a bottle of water for rehydration. You can even buy one with a handle for easy carrying!
- Let a family member or friend know the route you are taking.

YOUR WALKING PLAN

To start power walking you need to go three times a week, and you only need to do 20 minutes for each session. Plan your walk ahead of time so that you walk 10 minutes one way and 10 minutes back. That's how simple it is to start! You also need to introduce yourself to the six (see page xxx for details) basic body exercises to improve your general fitness.

When you start your first week of power walking, you need to walk at a speed that is just above your normal walking pace and is enough to make you feel you have pushed yourself. During your walk, it helps to hold your abdominal muscles in and work your arms in a forward and back motion, as this will work those abs and help tighten them up.

As you start your second week, it'll be time to start walking at a speed which will make you feel slightly out of breath. The best way to do this is to walk for 3 minutes at an easy pace, power up your speed for 1 minute and then return to an easy pace for 3 minutes to get your breathing back to its normal level.

Continue this each day until your breathing becomes easy and then you can slowly start increasing your power walking time and decreasing your walking time. Keep going until you can reach a full 20 minutes of power walking, at which point you should be feeling energised and good about what you have accomplished so far.

For week 3 continue power walking at a very brisk pace for the full 20 minutes. By now you should feel acclimatized to power walking. You've now completed your introduction to running and you are ready to start.

TIP

If you have a free day during the week, try taking an extra casual walk in your local park or countryside; just be sure to walk for at least 45 minutes.

HOW TO MAKE BREATHING EASY WHEN YOU RUN

Fact: When we run, we breathe harder. Running does involve a little bit of huffing and puffing; this is quite natural. For a newcomer to running it can be quite daunting to remember your running technique, focus on your running pace, and then concentrate on your breathing on top of everything—it can all feel quite overwhelming! Yet as the weeks go on, you will see that all the above things just fall naturally into place and you will do them all without even realising.

Most of us take shallow breaths when we run, which supplies our muscles with only a little oxygen, making running a little harder. Taking in a shallow breath whilst running is what fatigues us; more than our legs muscles feeling tired, it's the fact that we feel out of breath. Focusing on deeper breaths will help improve your endurance and your lung capacity.

Taking deeper breaths when you run is the key to making running easier; the more oxygen you take in when you run, the better the quality of breathing. This equals more oxygen for your muscles, and that equals more endurance, thus making running feel easier.

The first thing we need to do is to establish the difference between a shallow breath and a deep breath. As we know, we can breathe in through our nostrils and our mouth, but seeing that our mouth is far bigger than our nostrils, this is the way to take in that full deep breath.

Try this exercise to help your breathing: Start by taking a deep breath in as you walk, inhaling for three foot strikes, and then exhale for three foot strikes. This is known as deep breathing, as opposed to what is more likely what we have been doing (i.e., a shallow breath, in which you breathe in through the nose for just one foot strike and then out through the mouth for a foot strike).

This is a hard habit to break, and we can't expect to build Rome in a day. For beginners to running, this is a habit that we can start to form every week. If we can focus on taking the deeper breaths whilst we are walking then we have supplied the muscles with more oxygen for when we do the running intervals.

It is also a good habit to get into to always take ten deep breaths every day (let's call these belly breaths) as opposed to our normal breaths that we take all the time without even thinking (chest breaths).

So every day, while you are waiting for the kettle to boil or stuck at traffic lights, focus on doing ten deep belly breaths. Breathe in through your mouth for three counts, and then exhale by blowing out hard through your mouth for three counts. As you get more used to this, you can then increase this to five counts.

The great thing about deep breathing is that it helps improve your lung capacity and provides your muscles with more oxygen.

LISTEN TO YOUR BODY

No matter what form of exercise we do or what level we are at, it is highly important to listen to our bodies to prevent injury. Injury will interrupt your journey to getting fit, and consistency is the key to fitness.

- Never exercise on a full stomach.
- Never ignore medical conditions.
- Never compare yourself to others.
- Never exercise without stretching first.
- Never push yourself too hard.
- Stay hydrated.
- Stop if you experience pain or discomfort.
- Allow enough time for recovery.
- Never train with an injury.
- Never train when you have a cold or flu.
- Rest well and sleep well.

BEFORE YOU START

RUNNING TECHNIQUE TIPS

We are all individuals with our own unique method of running; therefore, there is no such thing as the perfect running style. Next time you see runners on TV, look at how each person runs quite differently, yet they are all still great runners. The following tips that I am going to share with you will allow you to perfect your own running style and get the most out of every stride you take.

Your height, weight and body shape will determine the length of your natural running stride. Your running stride and frequency determines how fast you run. This, simply, is why we all run differently. Let's break down the major body parts, so that when you are running you can focus on the right technique with these areas.

UPPER BODY

Keep your chest open, shoulders pulled back and down, chin parallel to the floor, and head facing forwards.

TUMMY

It is always important to keep your tummy muscles pulled in. This helps activate your deep core muscles which help maintain your good upper body posture.

LEGS

The main power of your running comes from your legs. You naturally engage your legs from your core muscles. A good visualisation is to imagine that strings are drawing your kneecaps forward as you run.

ARMS

Focus on them being bent at a 90-degree angle, and keep them relaxed as you move so they complement your natural running pace. The opposite arm to each leg should always move forwards.

HANDS

It is very easy to clench your fists while you are running but instead, focus on keeping them relaxed. Imagine that you are holding an eggshell between your thumb and forefinger without breaking it, so that your hands are still cupped without being clenched.

GROUND SURFACE

There are many types of ground surfaces to run on and each one will have its pros and cons. Training on uneven terrain like roads, sand or trails requires more body control and more balance, and it also activates more joints and muscles than working out on even, indoor surfaces.

ROADS AND PAVEMENTS

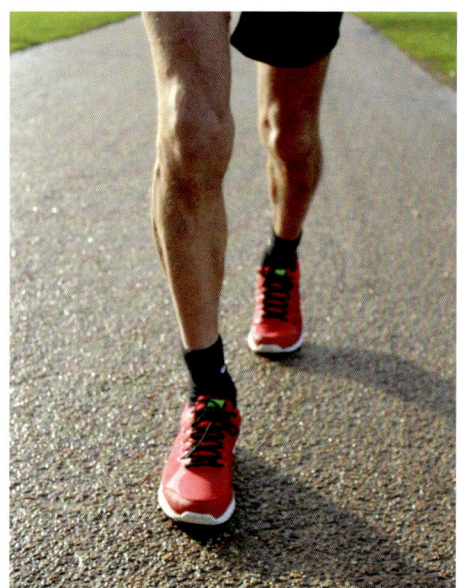

These are generally flat and accessible. The great feature of these is that you can plan your distance easier, they have lamp posts should you wish to add some speed training, and often there are benches where you can stop and stretch. However, these can be uneven and the risk of tripping on curbs at night is possible. Roads and pavements also give the most shock and impact to your joints and body, and the risk of injury is increased.

GRASSLAND

Park grasslands, football pitches and golf courses all offer soft ground to run on and work your muscles well. These are great places to run for beginners, although if you run on a golf course respect the golfers whilst they go about their business.

RUNNING TRACKS

These are fairly forgiving as they are always flat and absorb much of the shock of impact. Running tracks are a great place to work on your speed training as they are well marked to structure your intervals.

TRAIL RUNS

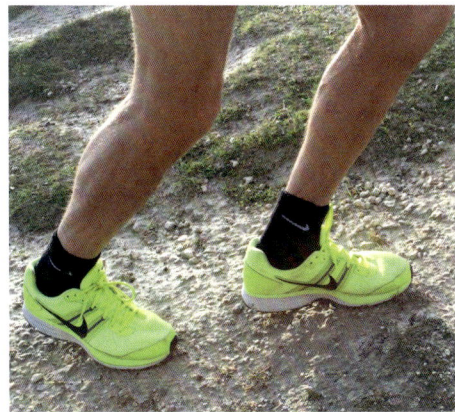

Trail running is often done through woodland and forests. It offers a much softer ground to run on and the ever-changing terrain makes this the number one choice for runners. With trail running, however, there are many natural obstacles to avoid so be careful of tree roots, rocks, over-hanging branches, etc.

BEACHES

Beaches can be a great place to run as the air is fresh and the scenery can be quite breathtaking. They are great places to build up strength in your legs, but you need to be very careful when running in very soft sand as there is a higher chance of injury.

HILL RUNNING

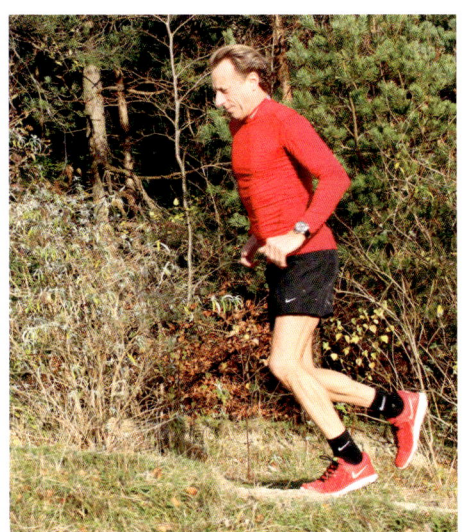

Hill running is one of my personal favourites as it's low impact and fires up all of the major muscles in your legs. Hill running is a great way to improve your stamina and will make you an overall better runner. But be warned, hills can be very tough and demanding!

YOUR FIRST RUN

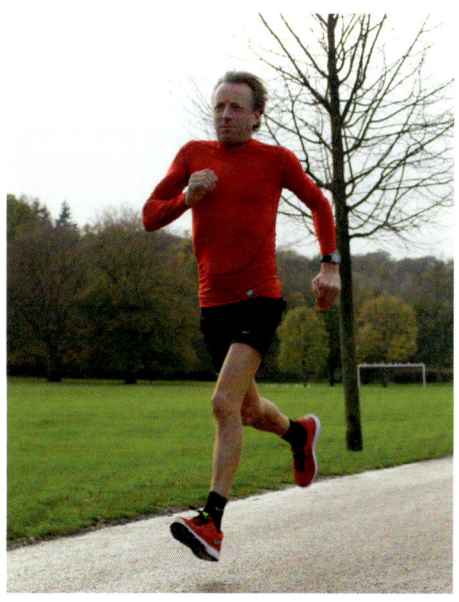

After completing your first three weeks of power walking you will have built up enough stamina and strength to progress onto running. You should now have faith in your body and be confident about taking your next step.

The first run can be tough, so be patient. The most important thing is to set yourself a very reasonable goal. You must run consistently right from the start and your body will soon acclimatise itself so that your following runs will get easier and the enjoyment will begin.

SETTING YOUR FIRST SMALL GOAL

When setting your first goal you need to make sure it's a reasonable goal. It should be something you know you can accomplish, as you do not want to disappoint yourself straight away. Your first goal should only be about time; you do not need to worry about speed, you just need to feel comfortable and you need to not push yourself too hard.

A fair goal to start with should be a time of 30 minutes and a target frequency of 3 times per week. It doesn't matter how far you run, it's just about running and walking for that time and slowly building up. It is important that you achieve your initial goal with a certain amount of ease so do not push yourself too hard, even if you are feeling good; just enjoy your first run. However, should you feel out of breath, tired or in any pain, then just walk.

You should finish your run with a great sense of achievement and be very proud of how far you have come.

UNDERSTANDING YOUR BODY

As you are new to running I will explain a little about what your body is going to feel. You will most probably feel tired after a run, and your muscles may ache, but worry not as this is a normal sensation for all runners at any level! Your body is not used to this movement and your muscle memory has forgotten what it is like to be used in this way. They will soon remember this new activity.

Within a couple of weeks your body will be much more accustomed to this level of activity and the more you run the easier it will get. During this period one of the best investments you can make is to have a sports massage. I have the most amazing therapist who helps me get my body back into shape and, to me, this is of paramount importance to my recovery and the prevention of injury. Another great investment is a foam roller, which will help to reduce any pain you are feeling with just a few simple exercises.

LONG-TERM GOALS

A reasonable ambition now is to be able to run the full 30 minutes nonstop. Again, this is just about being consistent and gradually building up your strength and stamina. It really doesn't matter how long it takes you to get up to this level, it's just about actually getting there free of injury and full of confidence.

Once you have more confidence and the ability to run a full 30 minutes, that is a good time to set yourself a goal of running your first race. If you are based in the UK, I would highly recommend Parkrun.com, a weekly 5K, free-entry, timed fun-run/jog for people of all ages. It is certainly a fun way to improve your running skill—once you have done your first run then your goal each week is to try for a PB (personal best)!

TIPS

- Take your time in building up your pace.
- Stay hydrated at all times.
- Listen to your body. If anything hurts, then slow down and walk.
- Make sure you stretch before and after each run.
- Try to run on grass or trails.
- If you run at night, wear a high-visibility jacket.
- Invite a friend to join you on your runs.
- Breathe easy and try to relax as you run.

HOW TO PROGRESS TO THE NEXT LEVEL

Now that you have built confidence levels, it is time to move forward and continue your progression. We need to look at making some small changes to start with. First, you now need to start increasing your running time; aim to do one longer run per week. Set yourself a goal that you are going to do a full hour run. Plan to do this at the weekend or whenever you have more time. Pick the route and terrain that suits you, preferably a trail run where there is no chance of boredom. Again, do not worry about how fast you run, just complete the time and feel tested.

MIX IT UP

Don't be afraid of doing things other than running. I like to cycle, as this is a great crossover into running. Cycling helps develop strength and is excellent for improving your overall aerobic strength. It is also a great way to avoid any injury as there is no impact, so try to include this as part of your training schedule.

PATIENCE

Never push yourself too hard as you increase your running. Injury prevention is crucial at this time as your body gets used to more stress, so never ignore a niggle or any on-going pain or discomfort as it will eventually get worse. Don't worry if achieving your training goals is taking longer than expected; it's just a matter of time and being consistent. Never do a big run without adequate recovery. After a long run, take time to eat, clean and refuel your body. Stretch or use a foam roller to release the tension and take a couple of days rest to recover well.

THE RUNNING TRACK

If you have now caught the running bug and doing a simple run or 5K race at an easy pace is not enough for you now is the time to add some high-quality speed work.

Speed training is without a doubt the most effective way to improve your running performance as you build strength in your leg muscles and increase the range of movement in your joints. It will also increase your capacity to produce energy very quickly and you will soon learn to relax whilst running at a much harder and faster pace.

Before you start, there are a few things to take into consideration, as these sessions will be very demanding:

- Warm up and cool down. Jog for at least 5 minutes to raise your temperature and increase blood flow to your muscles. After that do some gentle stretching and then revert to a gentle jog, adding some high knees and 20 metre sprints (though not flat out). Afterwards take a gentle jog and stretch again to cool down.
- Not too hard. An important rule to remember is that speed sessions are not all about running flat out until you are sick or about to pass out. They are about gradually increasing speed and improving your running form.
- Find a running partner. Speed work takes a lot of effort and willpower so having someone to train with will add focus and fun. And, if they are a faster runner than you, this will help push you harder.

There are many types of sessions you can do on a track. The ones I use are:

- Short bursts. These are running fast for a short period of time, and then taking as much time as you need to recover before starting again. For this type of training I use a marker of approximately 20 metres, run flat out, and then fully recover before I start again.
- Interval training. This is basically the same as short bursts except that the focus of this workout is to limit the rest period (interval) between each effort. The key to this type of training is that you do not fully recover between each effort.
- Using the 20-metre marker, your aim now is to run flat out to your finish point, then walk back to your start and set straight back off again. Aim to achieve 15 to 20 of these.
- Fartlek. Fartlek is a Swedish word for 'speed play' and this is the fun side of speed work as there are no set rules. Technically, it's not track training and is best done on roads, grass or trails. You simply mix bursts of hard running with periods of easy running. You just run fast bursts between trees, streetlights and parked cars just when you feel like it. You are your own boss on this.

Track workouts are very demanding on your body so be sure to treat them with respect. I believe one session every 2 weeks is more than enough to improve your speed. As with any type of hard training, recovery is the key so take it easy the day after.

HILL RUNNING

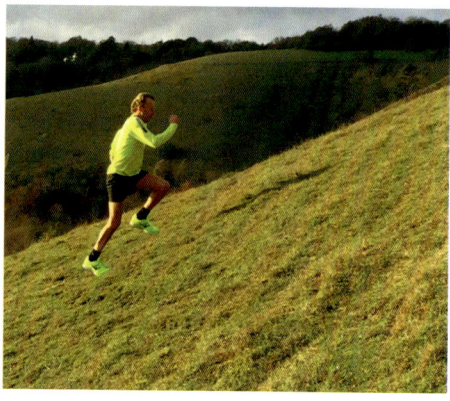

If you are now ready to test yourself on one of the toughest forms of training, then hill running has it all. Hill running will help you build stamina and will take your fitness to another level by greatly improving your leg muscles and lung function. You will engage everything from your lower legs to your hamstrings, hip flexors, core and lower back. Hill running is also a great way of minimising injury as there is less impact than you would normally get from pounding the ground.

Hill running promotes good running form because you are forced to get up on your forefoot, lift your knees, and drive your arms to propel yourself forward.

There are really two types of hills you should use in this training: the very steep to improve your endurance and the short incline for your speed work. With hill running you should try to include one of these disciplines every two weeks as your recovery time will take slightly longer. The result of hill running is you get fit fast!

HOW TO TACKLE THE STEEP HILL

For the best results, find a good, steep hill of about 400 metres that is set in the countryside or parkland and is a natural trail. Before you tackle the steep hill it is important that you have warmed up well, preferably by a short run of at least 15 minutes. This way your muscles will be warm and nicely stretched, but if you feel any pain during this exercise either stop or walk.

When taking on the steep hill make sure there is good footing so you do not slip. Set off and lean into the hill slightly as you run. This is not about speed, it's about just making it to the top! Keep your pace slow and try to control your breathing. Your heart will be pounding and it will feel like your chest will explode, but this is natural as you are pushing yourself to the extreme.

You will want to give up, your body will be saying 'No!' to this kind of punishment, but this is where visualisation comes in. Picture the top of the hill in your mind, visualise yourself conquering it, and feel the joy of your amazing achievement!

What works for me is just keeping my head down and watching my footing until I reach the top. When you have reached the top you should be completely breathless so try to walk it out and stretch your leg muscles. BE PROUD! You have just conquered your first hill!

SHORT HILL SPRINTS

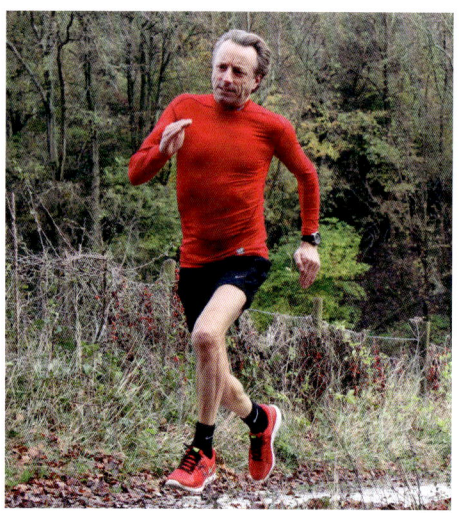

Short hill sprints are another great way to improve your running. As soon as you master this you will learn to be more relaxed when running at a much faster pace and be able to control your breathing more easily.

First, find yourself a good hill approximately 100 metres long. The hill should have a gradient of 6 to 8 percent with good footing. You will be powering your way up at full speed and you definitely don't want to slip.

With these short speed sprints you need to have some technique to apply. Your body will naturally lean into the hill, which is important in becoming a good sprinter. You will need to pump your arms much harder than normal, as this is where you will gain your power and momentum. You will also need to lift your knees a lot higher whilst sprinting.

HOW TO DO IT

You will need to work hard on this, as it will be tough; however, the training method is effective yet simple.

To start with you need to find some visible markers, which could be sticks or stones, and place one every 20 metres. These are going to be the points to which you run.

Before you start, make sure you have warmed up with a run and stretched well. The chances of injury are higher when sprinting, so stop if you feel any pain.

When you are ready to start, run at full speed to the 100-metre marker. Now take your time to walk back down to the start. Compose yourself and set off at full speed to the

80-metre marker. Again, head back down to the start and, when ready, run at full speed to the 60-metre marker, and so on.

Now take a short break to get your breathing under control and walk out any tightness in your legs. This exercise is tough so make sure you have some water on hand to hydrate yourself.

Now we reverse the discipline (20 metres, 40 metres, 60 metres, 80 metres, 100 metres) and that is your first set done. Repeat the entire exercise one more time and then take your time to cool down and stretch again.

You will eventually gain a great amount of confidence in hill running and learn to love this discipline just as I have done over time.

STAYING MOTIVATED

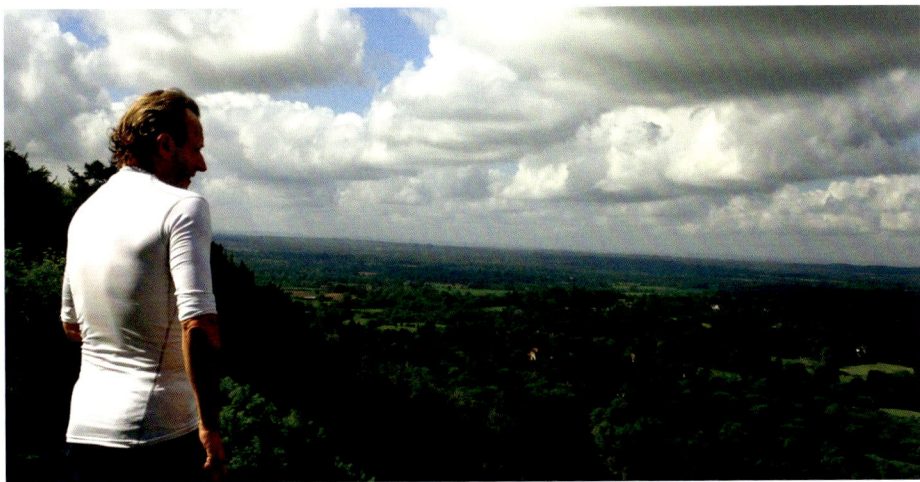

There will be times during your new training programme that you will begin to lose enthusiasm and question what you are doing. You may pick up an injury or miss a training run, and small things like this can make you feel like giving it all up. This is perfectly normal; even the best athletes have some self-doubt at times.

KEEP YOUR FOCUS ON THE POSITIVE

Keeping a list of all the things that you like about exercise can keep you focused. Examples might be:

- This is my personal time.
- The fresh air is good for me.
- I feel good and strong.
- I feel more confident about myself.

FIND A RUNNING BUDDY

Arrange to run with a friend, neighbour or work colleague at least once a week. This will keep you on track and help to eradicate any doubts. It is important to find someone who is around the same ability level and has the same energy and passion. This way you both help each other to remain focused and push yourself a little harder. It's a sure-fire way to never miss a training run!

KEEP A TRAINING LOG

A lot of runners (including myself) like to keep a training log. I find it helpful to review my weeks running. The easiest way is to design your own template that includes:

- The date
- Your mileage
- Your pace
- Your time
- How you felt during
- How you felt after
- Your route
- Off road or on

Keeping a training log will help to identify what works for you and what doesn't and will allow you to tweak your running programme to suit your needs.

DO A RACE FOR CHARITY

There is nothing better than committing yourself to doing a charity run. Your ideal start would be a 5K run as this is a fully achievable event at this early stage of your training. This will also give you the extra focus and challenge you need to commit yourself to your training programme. Once you have chosen the charity of your choice, collecting sponsorship money gives you another boost of determination.

USE MUSIC

If you enjoy listening to music then there can be nothing better than running to tracks that are uplifting and which can take your mind off fatigue during your run. However, you should always ensure that you can hear any other noise around you, especially if you are doing any road running.

REWARD YOURSELF

Now that you are following a regular training programme, your next level of goals should include rewarding yourself. Rewards may include buying a new addition to your training outfits. Nothing feels better than a new pair of running shoes or a new training top, and I find that if I feel good in the way I look, my training becomes much easier mentally.

RUNNING FAQS

Question: I find running so hard and just want to give up. What can I do to make it easier?

Answer: Try to focus on the two Rs: rhythm and relaxation. To get into a natural rhythm, concentrate on breathing in time with your feet as they strike the ground. Inhale as you take two strides, and then exhale fully as you take the next two strides. This helps you get that comfortable running pace and breathing rhythm. Now focus on relaxing into your run. Make sure you are not clenching your fists; check that your shoulders are relaxed and not hunched up by your ears; and just try and relax your body as you run. The more often you run, the more natural this becomes. The other element is to really focus on not running too fast or too slow. If you feel tired, go straight to a walking interval, get your breath back, and then take it back up again.

Question: I belong to a gym; should I use the treadmill or go running outdoors?

Answer: The best run will always be outdoors as it is you that is doing all the work and you have a much better variety of routes and terrain to run on. However, on a wet, miserable day a treadmill is a great option—and you can add a slight incline to make it tougher. But without a doubt, your best run will always be done outdoors, just try to stick to grass and trails.

Question: How do I get started with running?

Answer: The best way to do it is in small steps, and this is why I have devised this programme in which, week by week, you become fitter and more adapted to running. Start with walking and small intervals of running. Then each week as you become fitter and your body becomes more relaxed with running, increase the running intervals so you progress naturally, and you will see how easy running can be.

Question: Can I run if I have a cold?

Answer: I can only give you my best advice. If you have a runny nose or sore throat and are just feeling a little run down then, yes, just take a gentle run and do not push yourself too hard. If, however, you have a chesty cough and flu-like symptoms, then I suggest that you rest and wait until you have fully recovered.

Question: I am worried that if I start running I will become very hungry. Is there a danger that I will start overeating?

Answer: This is a common myth, but the answer is no, not at all. Simply put, the more exercise your body does the more calories you burn. If you feel hungry after a run, the important thing is to make sure that you eat the right snack. Avoid processed foods, and stick with the sort of snack options here in this book. It is also important to stay fully hydrated. Dehydration can sometimes be confused with hunger, so always keep those water levels topped up. You do not need to worry about weight gain.

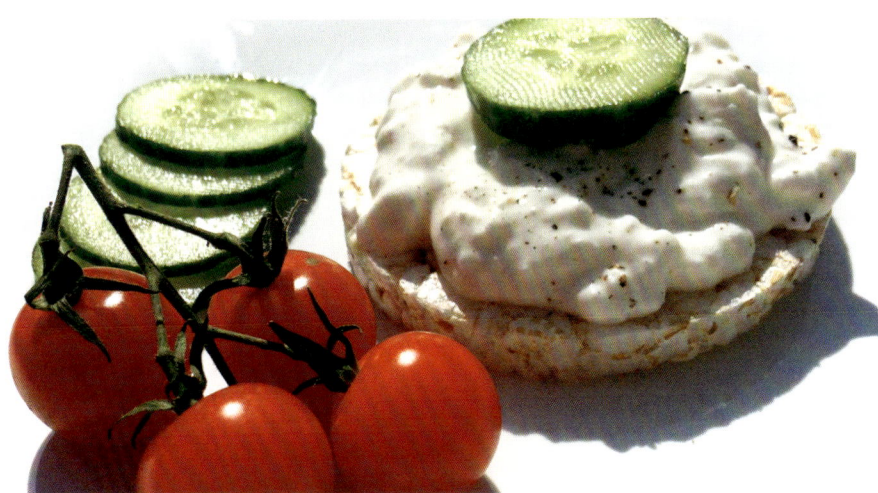

Question: What is a recovery run?

Answer: A recovery run is a slow, light run to help your body recover from any hard training sessions you have done. As this is a recovery, just take a very gentle 15-minute jog to ease any tight muscles.

Question: I am 59 years old. Am I too old to start exercising?

Answer: Absolutely not! You are never too old to exercise, just be sure to consult with your doctor first. If you have no known medical conditions, start slowly and gradually build up in intensity. Most importantly, do not over-train or over-stretch. Listen to your body!

Question: What is the best time to go for my run?

Answer: This is down to each individual. If you are a morning person, then set the alarm early and head off before work, but always make sure you have enough time to stretch and warm up properly beforehand. Personally, I prefer to run in the evenings in the winter and early mornings in the summer.

RUNNING FUEL

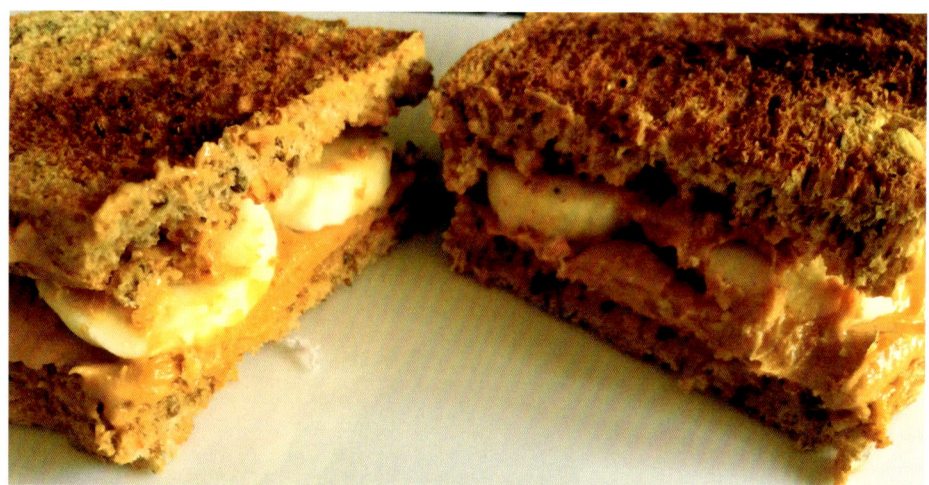

A question we all ask ourselves is 'What is the ideal food to eat to accompany our running?' You will find that most runners will give you the same answer: pasta. This may be the runner's ideal choice as it's a starchy carbohydrate which fuels your body for your runs, and it will give you a slow-release of energy, particularly if you are covering long distances. However, pasta alone cannot fuel your balanced running diet.

Due to the demands that running puts on your body it is just as important to include good quality protein such as lean meat, fish, dairy, eggs and pulses to help repair, build and ensure that your muscles are kept in the best possible condition.

Most people who take up running for weight loss overlook fats. Good fats provide a necessary source of energy and vitamins for your body. These can be found in oily fish, nuts, seeds, olives and avocados.

Fruits and vegetables also play a very important role in your running fuel. Everybody should focus on five portions per day but as a runner your energy and nutritional demands will be higher. Select vegetables like broccoli, kale, cabbage, peppers and carrots every day as these contain high amounts of nutrients.

Your legs will take a huge amount of pounding from a high-impact sport such as running. The soreness you often feel after a hard training session is partly caused by micro tears in your leg muscles, so berries (and their high fibre content), vitamin C and potassium play an important part in helping to repair your body.

Water, though technically not a food, is a vital part of your running fuel so stay hydrated at all times.

A healthy and well-balanced combination of carbohydrates, protein, fats and fluids is necessary for your body to become a good and efficient runner.

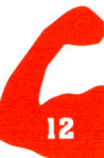

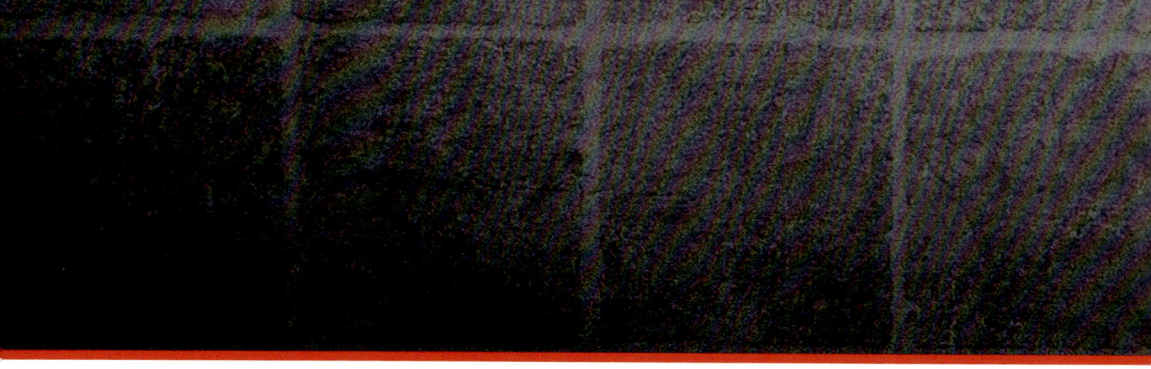

13 EXERCISE

There comes a time for all of us when we feel that life is catching us up, and we begin to feel a pressing need to get fit for personal or health reasons. The question is: Where do we start?

We look at fitness magazines, but it is sometimes difficult to relate to the young fitness models with six packs, huge chests and bulging biceps. Gyms are expensive and invariably busy, and can be intimidating for some of us.

Running strengthens your muscles and gives you a feeling of general fitness, but you also need to include some sophisticated resistance workouts to improve your overall body composition.

I will share with you my secrets for building your body, and show you some amazing indoor and outdoor body weight and resistance workouts.

BECOME YOUR OWN GYM

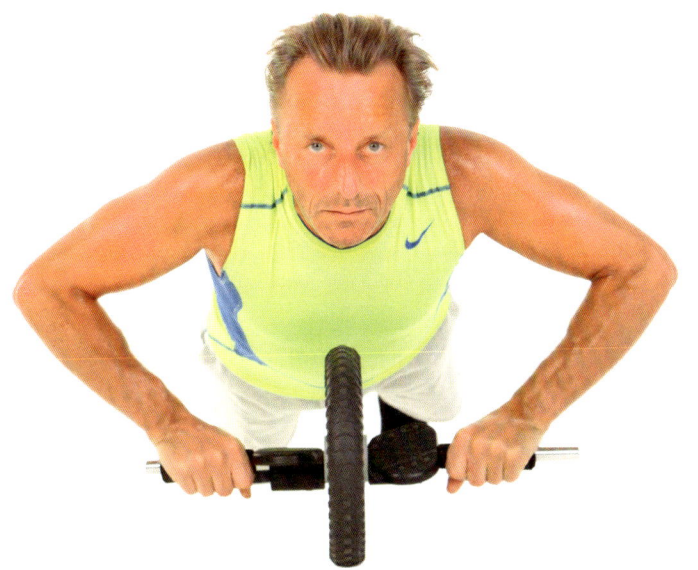

To complement your running and overall fitness, there are five basic indoor exercises to start with. These are simple yet powerful moves which will tone and strengthen your body and also improve your running skills. Although they can be done indoors, performing these exercises in your local park where the air is fresh and nature is all around is even better for you!

If you are a complete beginner to exercise, always check with your doctor before you start any new exercise programme.

LUNGE

The lunge is a body resistance exercise that works the leg muscles specifically. It targets the quadriceps and the hamstring muscles in the thighs, and the gluteal muscles in the buttock and the lower leg muscles.

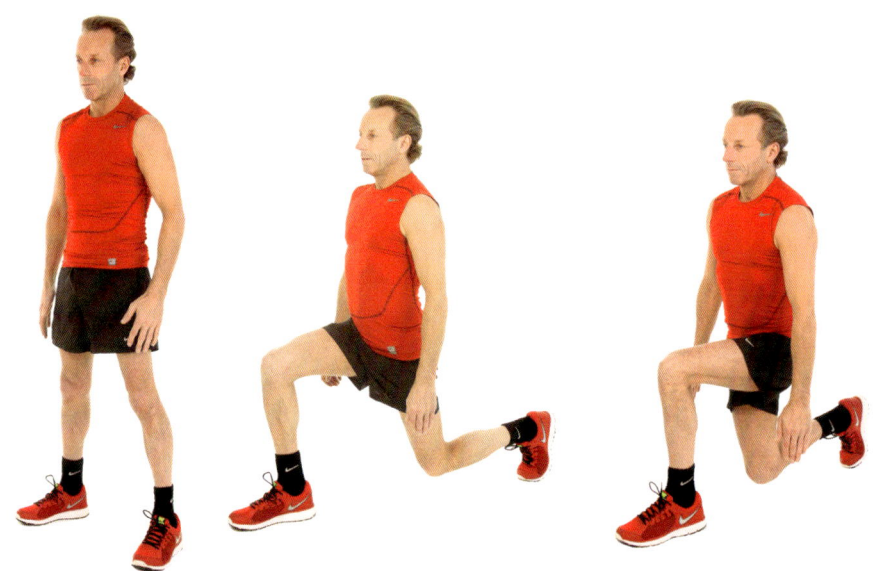

INSTRUCTIONS

- From a standing position, step forward with one leg, lowering your hips until both knees are bent at a 90-degree angle.
- Make sure your front knee is above your ankle and does not extend past your toes.
- Make sure your other knee doesn't touch the floor.
- Keeping your weight in your heels, push back to the starting position.
- Do 15 reps with each leg.

SQUAT

The squat is a compound, full-body exercise that primarily trains the thighs, hips, buttocks, quadriceps and hamstrings. The squat also works the core, and improves balance and coordination.

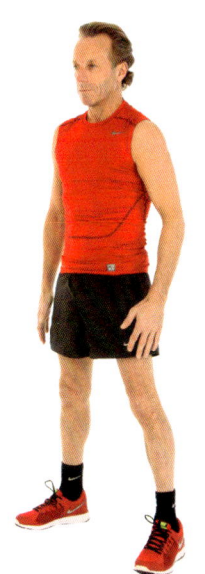
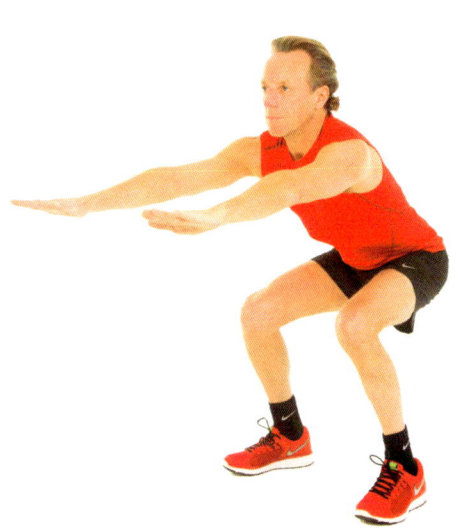

INSTRUCTIONS

- Stand with your feet a little wider than shoulder-width apart.
- Extend your arms straight out with your palms facing down.
- Bend your knees, place your weight over your heels, and sit down as though you are sitting in a chair.
- Keep your chest forward and head up.
- Press through your heels back to the start position.
- Start with 15 reps every day, and slowly build up to more.

PRESS-UP

The press-up exercises the major muscle groups, the chest and triceps. It also engages every muscle between the shoulders and toes, including all the important core muscles in the abdomen. Press-ups are a great exercise, and there are many variations you can do to improve your overall physique.

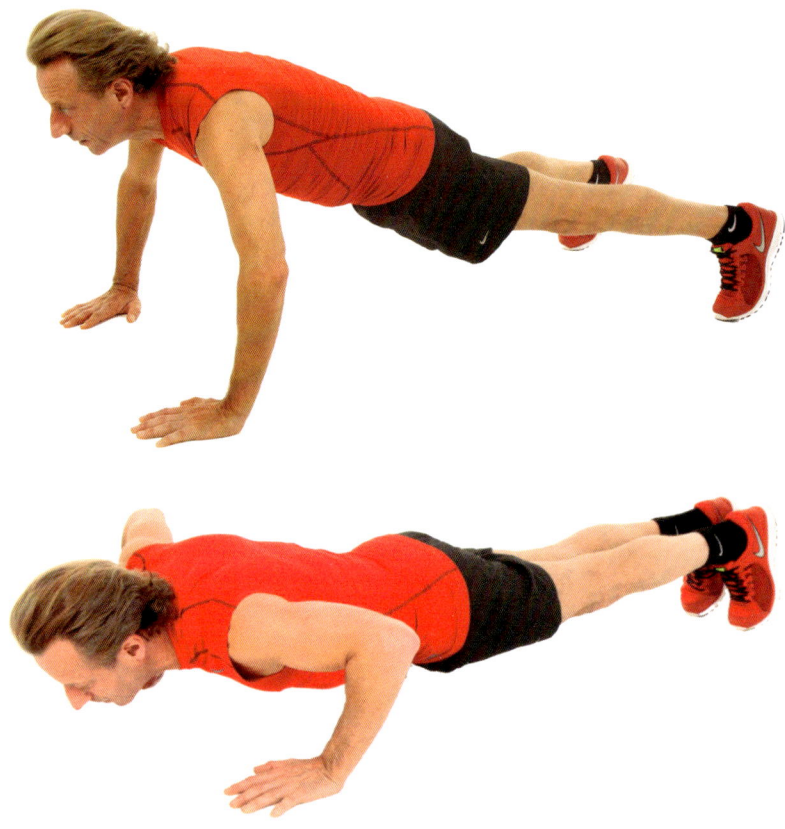

INSTRUCTIONS

- Get into the plank position with hands slightly wider than shoulder-width apart.
- Keep your feet together and ground your toes to stabilize the bottom half of your body.
- Engage your abs and slowly lower yourself to the floor, keeping your back flat and your neck straight.

- Don't let your butt dip or stick up during this move; your body should remain straight.
- Keep the elbows tucked close to the body so the upper arms form a 45-degree angle at the bottom of the move.
- Keeping your core muscles engaged, exhale and press back up to your starting position.
- Start with 15 reps every day, and slowly build up to more.

ABDOMINAL CRUNCH

The abdominal crunch is a great exercise to help strengthen, tone and stabilize the muscles of the core, particularly the rectus abdominis. It also targets the oblique muscles which run down the sides of your abdomen.

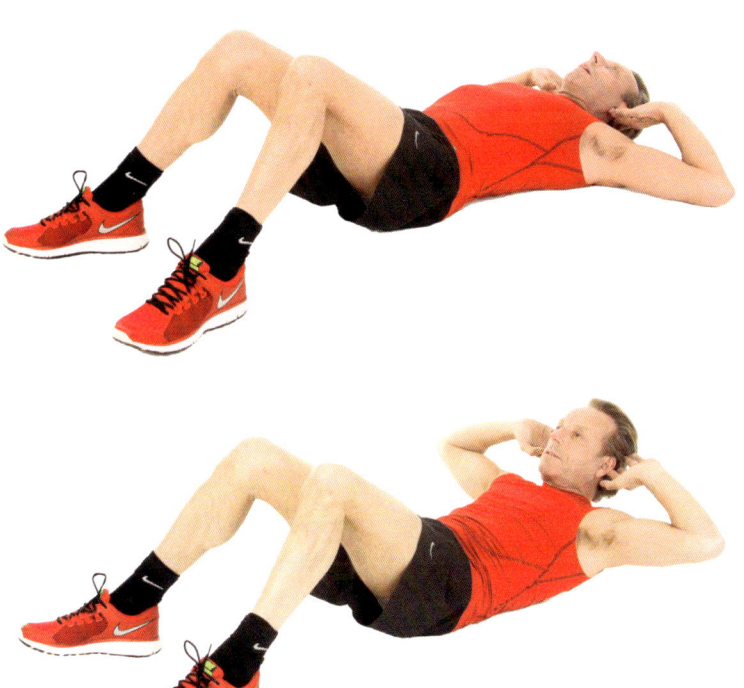

INSTRUCTIONS

- Lie down on the floor on your back and bend your knees. Place your hands behind your head or across your chest.
- Pull your belly button toward your spine, and keep your lower back flat to the floor.
- Contract your abdominal muscles, bringing your shoulder blades several inches off the floor.
- Exhale as you come up, keeping your neck straight and your chin up.
- Hold at the top of the movement for just a few seconds.
- Slowly lower yourself back down, but do not relax all the way down.
- Do 20 reps while keeping your form good.

THE FOREARM PLANK

The forearm plank is one of the best exercises you can do to work hard on your core muscles. This is a very simple exercise, but with good technique it will help build your isometric strength, build your waistline and improve your posture.

INSTRUCTIONS

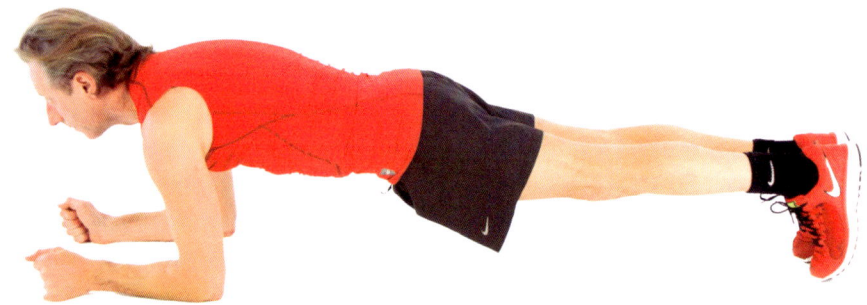

- Lie facedown with your legs fully extended.
- Rest your forearms on the ground with your elbows aligned below your shoulders.
- Keep your arms parallel to your body about shoulder-width apart.
- Keep your hands flat on the floor.
- Straighten your body, keeping your neck and spine in a neutral position.
- Hold this position for 1 minute to start with and gradually build up your time.

THE SIDE PLANK

This is a variation of the forearm plank which engages your obliques.

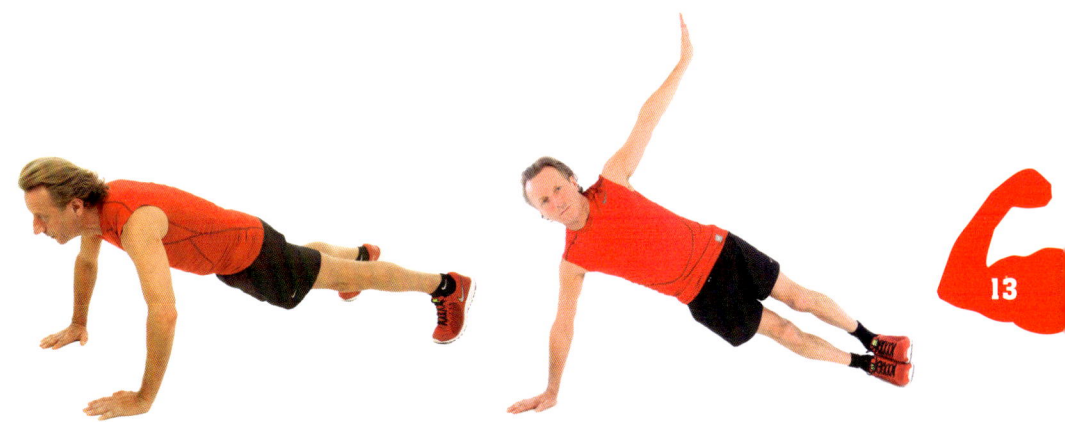

INSTRUCTIONS

- Lie on one side with one leg on top of the other.
- Raise your body up with your weight on your arm.
- Keep your feet on top of each other.
- Raise your opposing arm into the air keeping it parallel to the other.
- Hold this position for 1 minute to start with and gradually build up your time. Repeat on the other side.

SKIPPING

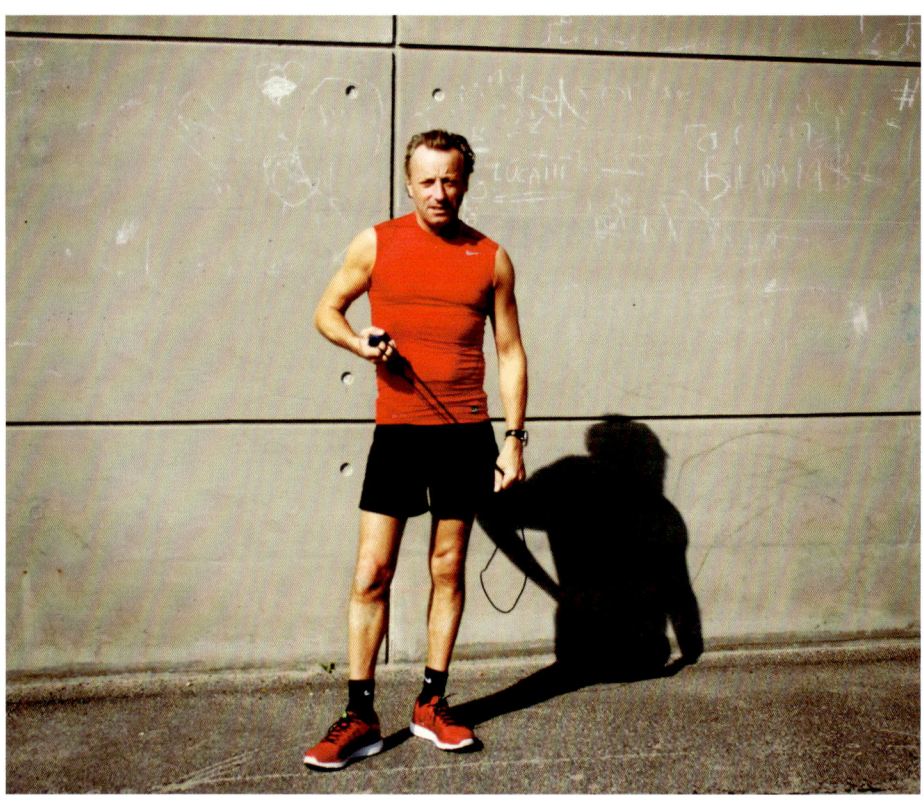

Skipping gets your heart rate up very quickly, so if you have been leading a sedentary lifestyle you should check with your doctor that you are fit enough to start an exercise program. Begin by skipping for 20 to 30 seconds, then march in place for 30 seconds. Repeat for 10 minutes. As your fitness level improves, increase the length of time skipping.

Your heart is the most important muscle in your body and needs regular exercise to stay strong and healthy. Skipping is one of the simplest and best ways to exercise your heart.

The stronger your heart becomes, the fitter you feel. You'll feel less breathless when you work out, and each day you will have heaps more energy if you include this in your training plan.

You can include skipping with all the above exercise and get a full-body workout. Initially you should try skipping for just 1 minute before moving on to the exercises. As you get fitter, increase the minutes you skip and the number of reps of each exercise. Trust me, in time you will get fitter and healthier, so don't SKIP those workouts!

14 THE ULTIMATE OUTDOOR WORKOUTS

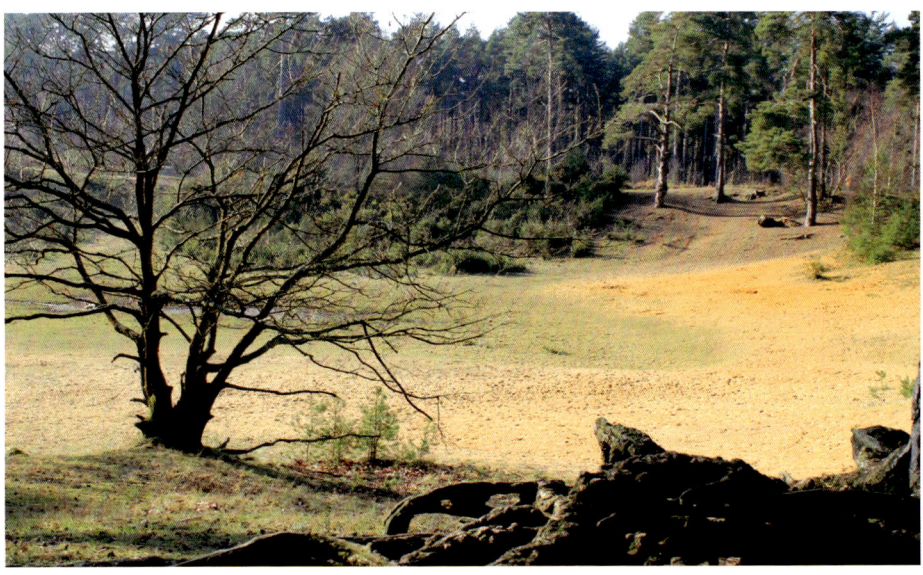

For me there really is only one way to work out and that is being outdoors. I personally couldn't think of anything worse than training in a gym which is expensive and full of smelly, stale air and full-grown men grunting and strutting their stuff. It can be very intimidating! So stop ignoring your instincts—nature is the perfect training ground and it's free and open 24 hours a day. The varied terrain of the outdoors is what your body needs to challenge itself to move in a more complex way. You can build muscle just as effectively using your own body weight as you can by lifting iron weights.

All you need is a little imagination and something that you can push, pull and lift. You may have rain, wind and hot weather to contend with so your body will work so much harder to compete with the conditions.

HOW TO GET STRONGER WITH A LOG

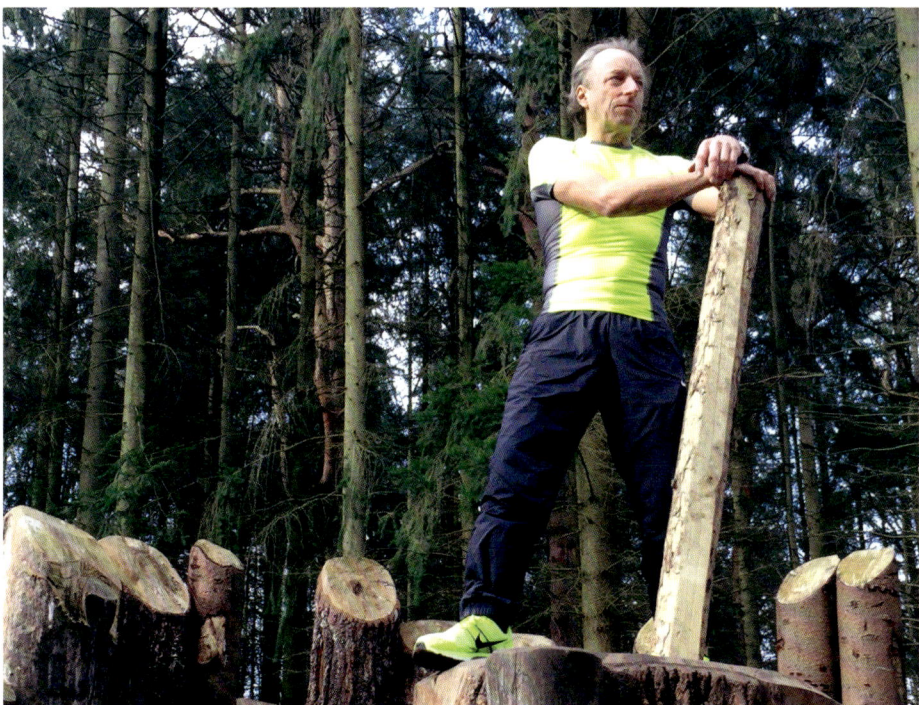

This workout focuses on strengthening all the key areas of your chest, back, abs, arms and legs. For me, training with a log has many benefits. There is no need to invest in weights or equipment; you just head to the woods and find a log. The log encourages you to use certain moves and to travel through a vast range of movements. As you get stronger, simply find a bigger log. The length of the log also allows you to take a wider grip which is great for ensuring we target all of the muscle groups to reach their full potential.

BEFORE YOU START

As with any workout, always ensure you have warmed up properly to prevent any injuries and perform your exercises efficiently and more effectively.

For this workout, it may be a good idea to wear some gloves to avoid getting any splinters. Make sure your gloves provide a good grip. Now, find your log and let's get started!

EXERCISE 1: LATERAL LOG DROP

The lateral log drop is a great way to strengthen the muscles on the inside and outside of your thighs, known as the abductors and the adductors. These muscles are often neglected in training as we tend to focus more on the front and back muscles, and these get engaged as you lower the log from side to side. Not only will this build power in your legs but it will also help prevent knee injuries. The stronger these muscles are the more support your knees have.

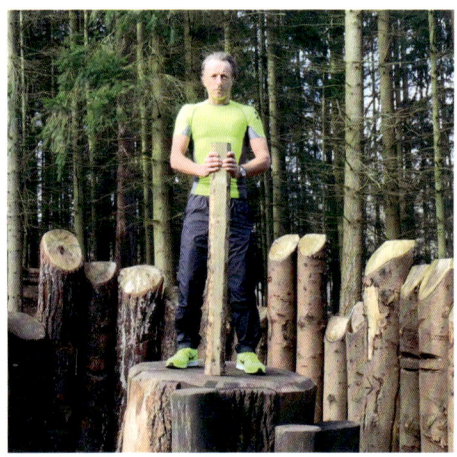
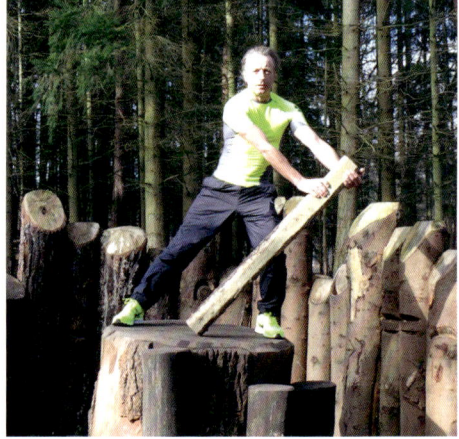

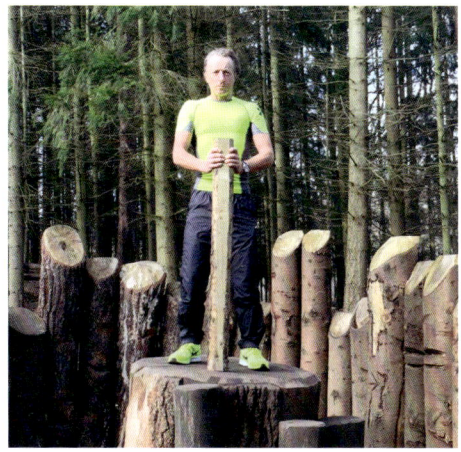 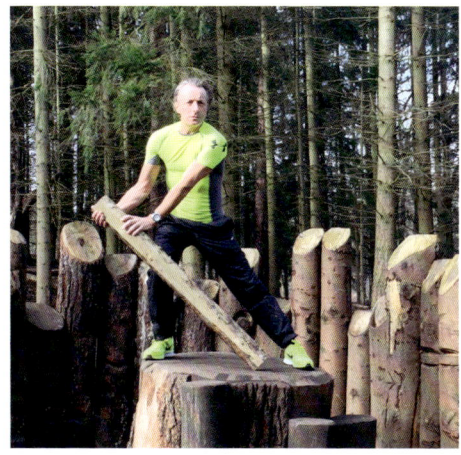 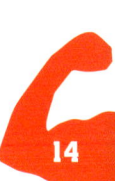

INSTRUCTIONS

- Stand with good posture with the log upright and with your hands gripping either side of it.
- Slowly lunge one leg out to the side as if you're aiming to take the log toward either an 11 o'clock or 2 o'clock position.
- Hold this position for a couple of seconds then push straight back to your start position.
- Repeat the exercise to other side.
- 5. Perform 20 reps 3sets

TIP

As you get fitter you can aim to take the log to a lower point such as a 9 o'clock or 3 o'clock position.

EXERCISE 2: THE BICEPS CURL

This is one of the most familiar and basic exercises you can perform. It's great for targeting and building strength in your upper arms.

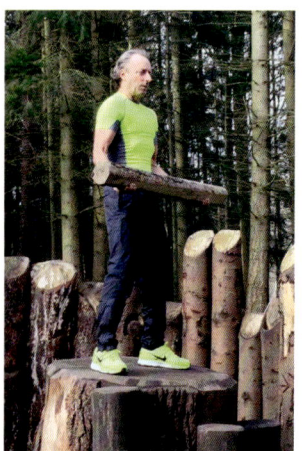
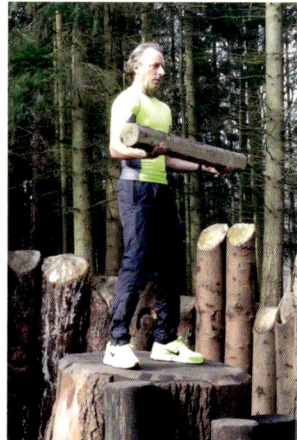
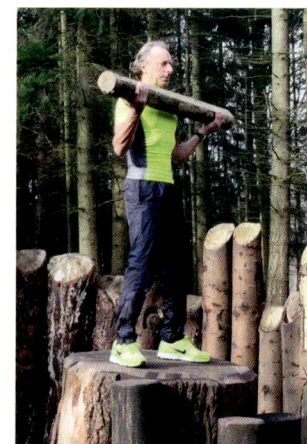

INSTRUCTIONS

- Stand with your feet hip-width apart and hands shoulder-width apart.
- Let your arms hang straight down with your palms facing up with the log resting in them. Your elbows should be close to your torso.
- Draw in the tummy muscles as you slowly curl your arms up until the log is in front of your chest.
- Slowly lower the log back to the start position.
- Perform 3 sets of 20 reps each.

EXERCISE 3: THE LOG AB TWIST

This move specifically targets your internal and external oblique muscles, which will help develop a strong chiselled six pack. In order to work your arms more you can hold the log further away from your body so that your arms have to do more work.

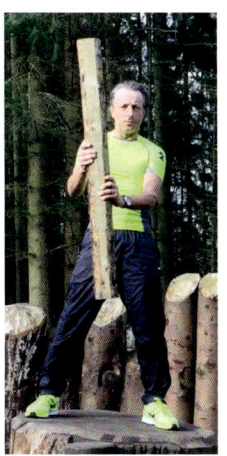
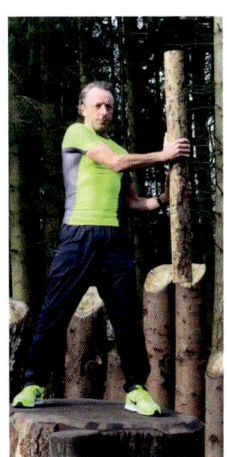
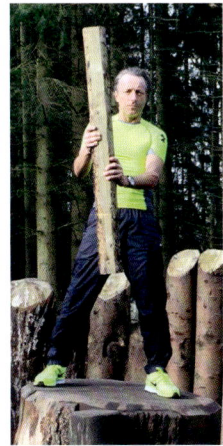
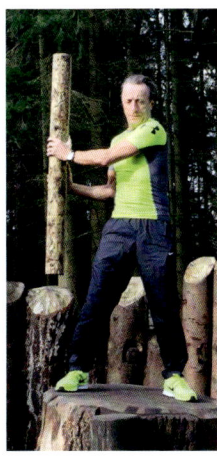

INSTRUCTIONS

- Hold your log in a vertical position with a firm grip in the centre. Stand with your feet hip-width apart, your knees slightly bent and your hips facing forward.
- In a controlled movement, slowly rotate the log around to one side, making sure you do not twist from the hips.
- Hold at the furthest point for a few seconds, slowly come back to the centre, and then rotate around to the opposite side.
- It is important you do not move the hips so imagine they are set in concrete. This ensures you are targeting your oblique muscles and working on building your six pack.
- Perform 3 sets of 12 reps each.

EXERCISE 4: THE LOG SQUAT

This move is one of the best ways to quickly build strength and power in your lower body. Traditionally, the squat is a must in any routine. Here we give it even more of a challenge by adding a log, which creates more resistance so you have to work your glutes and hamstrings harder as you push back up.

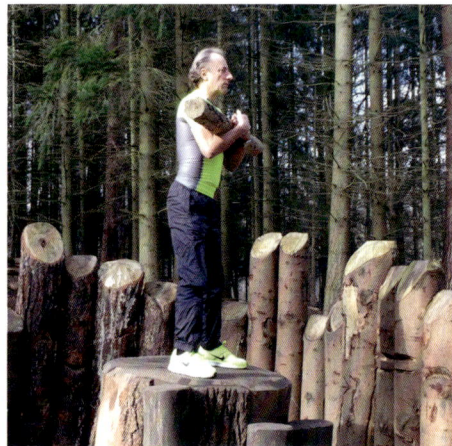 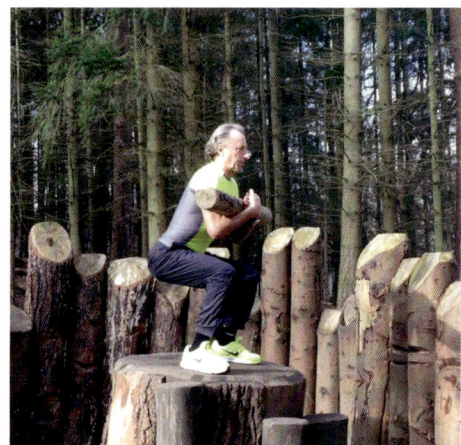

INSTRUCTIONS

- Start with your feet hip-width apart.
- Make sure you have the log gripped closely to your chest with your arms crossed.
- Keeping the log to your chest, slowly bend through the knees as if you are about to sit down. Make sure you do not let your knees go beyond your toes.
- Hold the position for a couple of seconds then slowly push back up to your start position.
- Perform 3 sets of 20 reps each.

EXERCISE 5: THE LOG OVERHEAD PRESS

This exercise works your shoulders and arms and naturally engages deep into your core muscles. By taking a wider grip, you also engage your lats (the big muscles on your back) and help build that lean, strong, chiselled look.

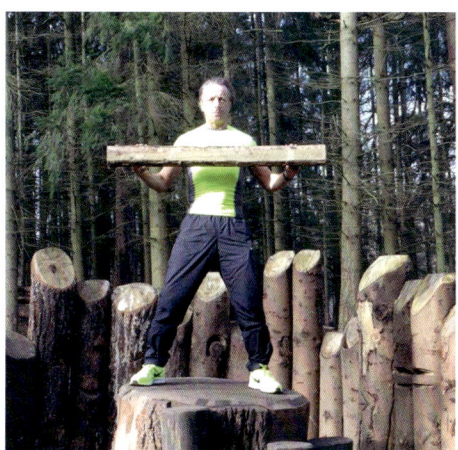
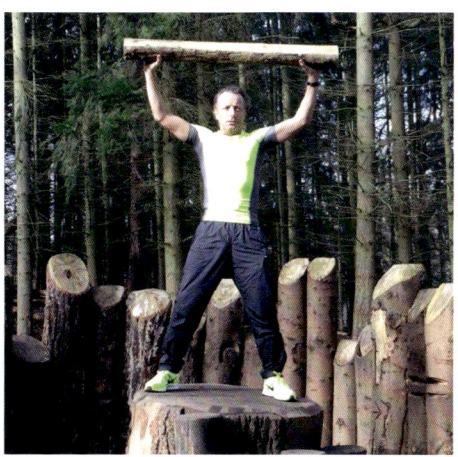

INSTRUCTIONS

- Start with your feet slightly wider than shoulder-width apart.
- Have your hands at either end of the log with your palms facing forward, ensuring you have a good grip of the log.
- Pull your tummy muscles in tight, and then slowly lift the log directly above and slightly in front of your head.
- Hold for a few seconds and then slowly lower it back down to your starting position.
- Perform 3 sets of 12 reps each.

EXERCISE 6: THE LUNGE AND BICEPS CURL

With this exercise you get double the benefits as the lunge works your entire lower body and the biceps curl helps build muscles and strengthen the arms. This exercise also engages your motor skills, thereby developing better coordination. It is a great way to help keep your nervous system strong.

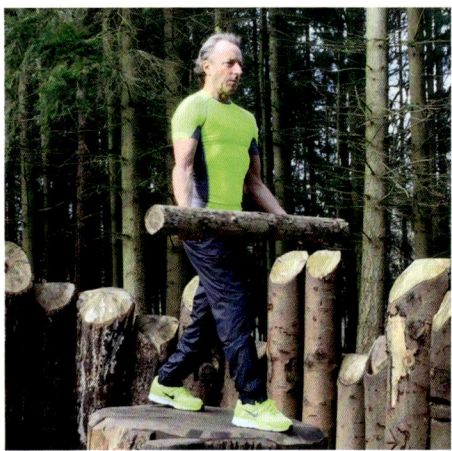
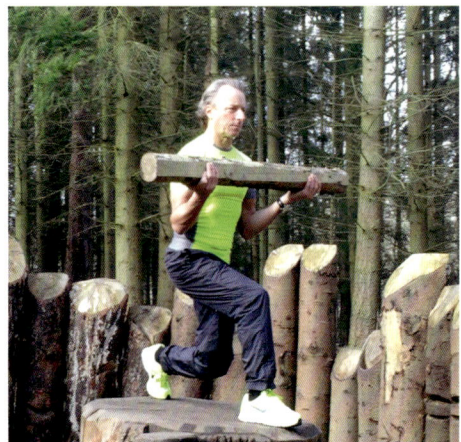

INSTRUCTIONS

- Step one foot forward into a split lunge stance. Holding onto the log with your palms facing up and hands shoulder-width apart, engage your abs.
- Slowly bend your knees, lowering them behind you toward the ground while, at the same time, bringing the log up toward your chest.
- Hold this position for a couple of seconds, then slowly come up to your start position.
- Do 10 reps on each leg; 3 sets.

TIP

As you get fitter you can increase the amount of reps and then when you are ready move up to the next size log.

THE SANDBAG WORKOUT

This workout is a winner for a number of reasons. You can do this in your back garden and there is no need to buy expensive equipment. Just pop down to your local garden centre and pick up a hessian sandbag and a bag of sand.

The following workouts are designed using only a simple sandbag which you are going to grab, drag and pull. The exercises are heavy duty enough to last you for a good few months!

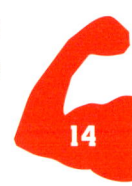

EXERCISE 1: THE SANDBAG PULL

This move works the muscles located at the back of your upper arms, known as the triceps.

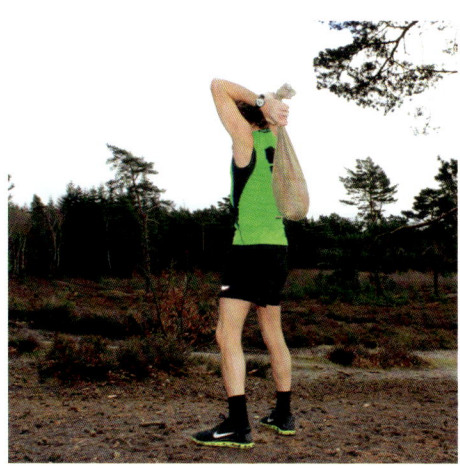
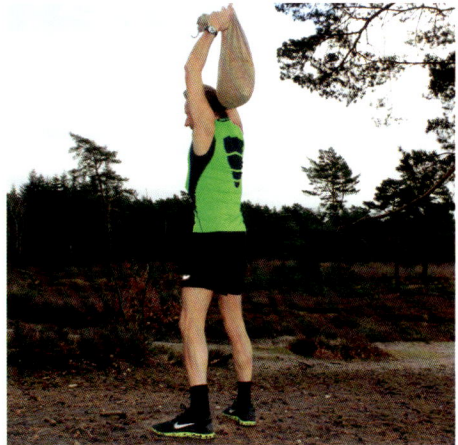

INSTRUCTIONS

- Stand with your feet hip-width apart, knees soft, and abs pulled in. Hold the sandbag behind you with both hands and a firm grip.
- Start with your elbows bent, then slowly extend your arms so they are straight, lifting the sandbag up your back.
- When your arms are fully extended, hold that position for a second, then slowly lower your arms back to your start position.
- Perform 3 sets of 12 reps each.

EXERCISE 2: THE SANDBAG ROW

This exercise will mainly work your chest, back and biceps muscles in a controlled isolated movement.

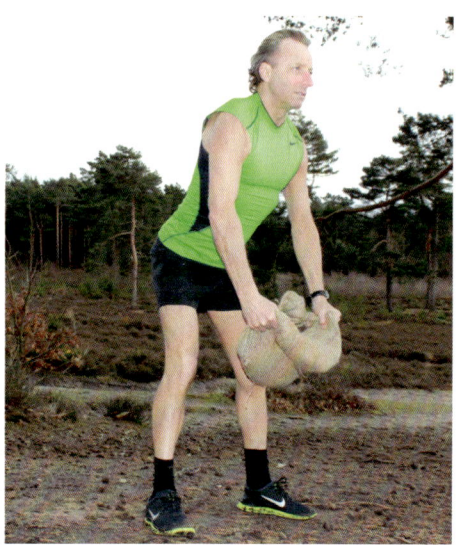
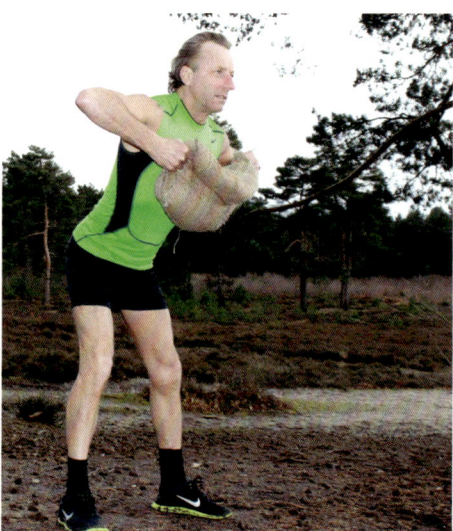

INSTRUCTIONS

- Stand with your feet hip-width apart and knees slightly bent. Lean forward with your chest over your feet, arms down and holding the sandbag at each end.
- Slowly bring the sandbag tight up to your chest and then back to the start position.
- Perform 3 sets of 15 reps each.

EXERCISE 3: THE SANDBAG SWING

This move engages both your lower body and upper body at the same time and is great for building power and strength in your legs, abs, shoulders and arms.

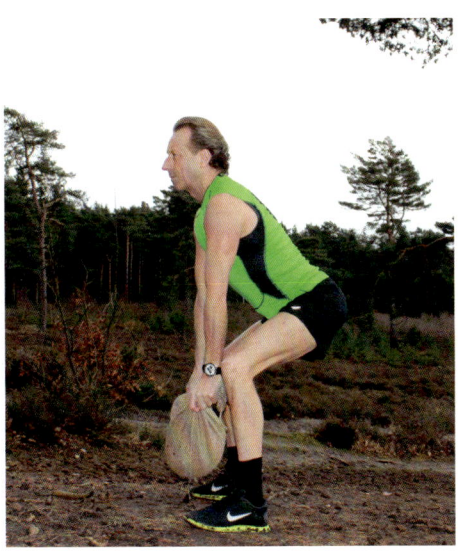 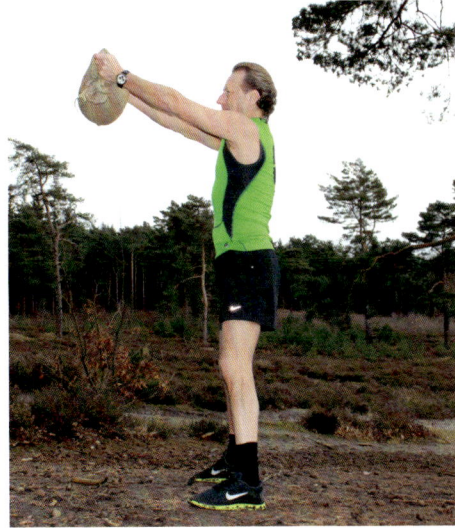

INSTRUCTIONS

- Start in a squat position, holding onto the sandbag with a firm grip.
- In a quick and controlled motion, come up to standing and, at the same time, swing the sandbag up to shoulder height. Then move straight back to your squat position.
- Keep your abdominal muscles engaged throughout this move.
- Perform 3 sets of 20 reps each.

EXERCISE 4: THE SANDBAG SQUAT JUMP

The sandbag squat jump is a compound, full-body exercise that trains the thighs, hips, buttocks, quadriceps and hamstrings. The squat also works the core and improves balance and coordination.

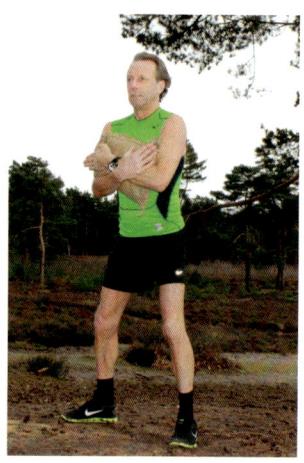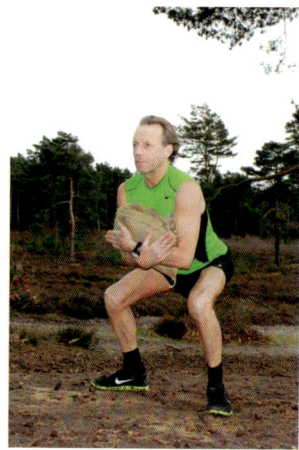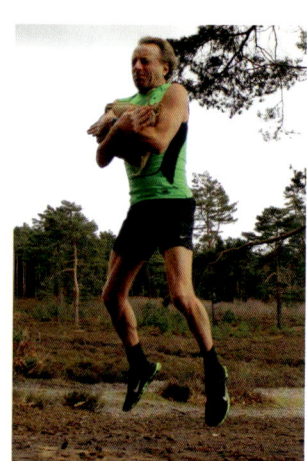

INSTRUCTIONS

- Stand in an upright position with your feet a little wider than shoulder-width apart and your knees slightly bent. Keep the sandbag close to your chest and your arms crossed.
- Slowly bend down into a squat position with your weight over your heels.
- In one powerful move explode upward and land back in the squat position again.
- Perform 2 sets of 10 reps each.

EXERCISE 5: THE SANDBAG DRAG

This exercise works your lateral muscles and builds strength in your arms, chest and shoulders, all while giving your entire abdominal muscle group an intense workout. You engage these muscles to help stabilize yourself as you drag the bag from side to side.

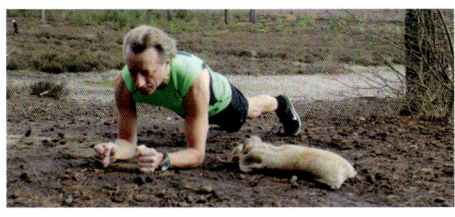
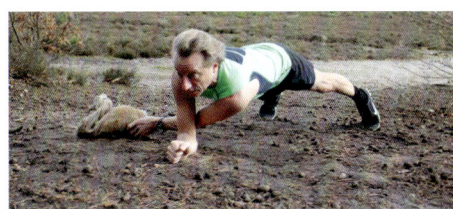

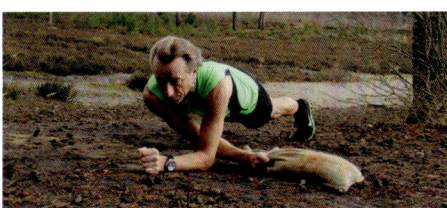
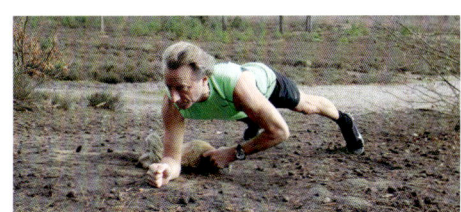
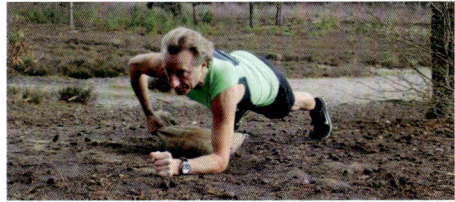
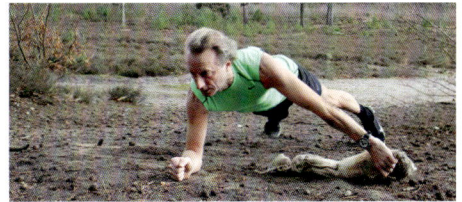
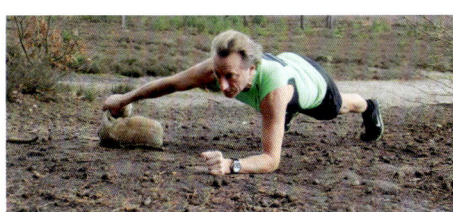

INSTRUCTIONS

- Starting in a plank position with the sandbag on the ground out to your left side, reach your right arm under yourself to grab the bag and pull it out to your right side.
- Repeat the exercise, this time using your left hand to pull the bag from your right side.
- Perform 3 sets of 10 reps each.

EXERCISE 6: THE SANDBAG AB TWIST

This move specifically targets your internal and external oblique muscles by challenging your torso muscles from every angle.

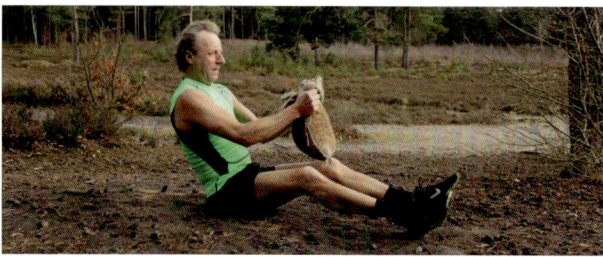

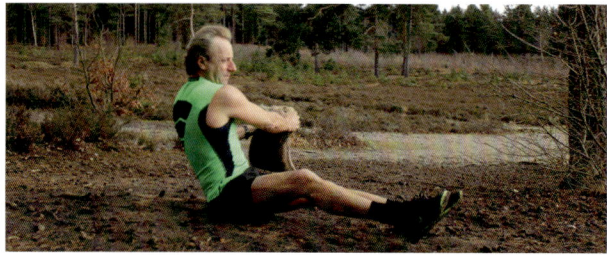

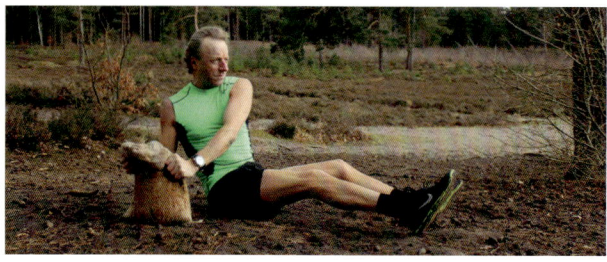

INSTRUCTIONS

- In a seated position with your feet hip-width apart and your knees slightly bent, hold the sandbag at chest height.
- In a controlled movement, slowly rotate the sandbag around to one side, making sure you do not twist from the hips.
- Hold for a few seconds at the furthest point, and then slowly come back to the centre and rotate around to the opposite side.
- Perform 3 sets of 10 reps each.

THE STAIR WORKOUT

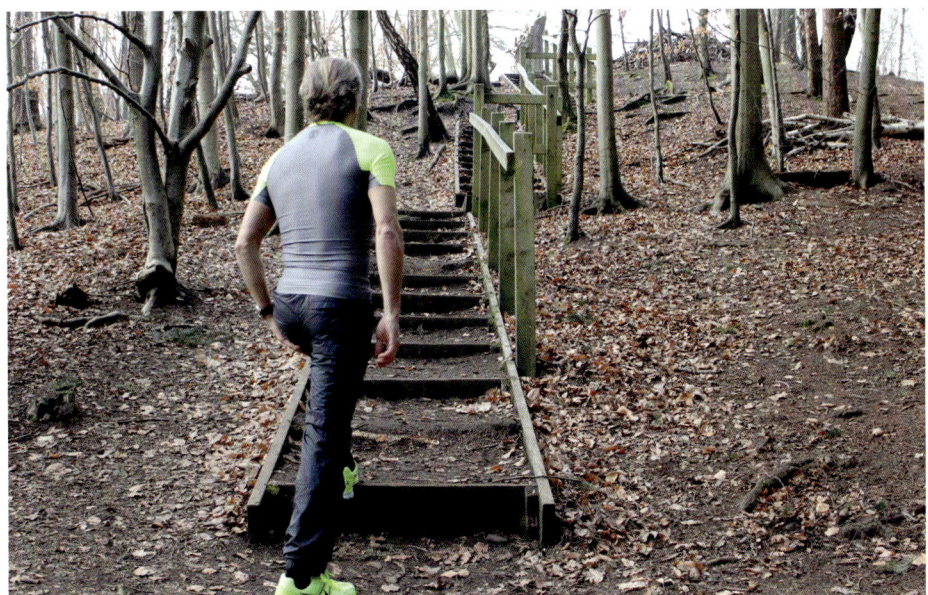

A stair workout is an incredibly effective way to improve your fitness and overall health. Stairs are a simple yet amazing piece of equipment. It's not always easy to find stairs in the outdoors, but once found they will become an important part of your training ritual. Outdoor steps may be cut into the natural terrain, may be different widths, and may be of varying heights; these differences can make your routine far more challenging and more varied.

There are many exercises you can do on a set of stairs, from just running to a complete body workout where you can undertake a full range of movements engaging more muscle groups. These exercises create a powerful cardio workout which will crank up your heart rate and help you burn fat.

Prior to starting the stair workout make sure you are fully warmed up. Depending on how long the stairs are, make a marker for your start and finish; give yourself an achievable amount of steps to accomplish, but do not over-stretch yourself.

EXERCISE 1: CROSS-STEPS

Cross-steps work your lateral leg muscles. These muscles are often neglected as we mainly use a forward and backward motion, which strengthens your quadriceps and your hamstrings (your front and back leg muscles).

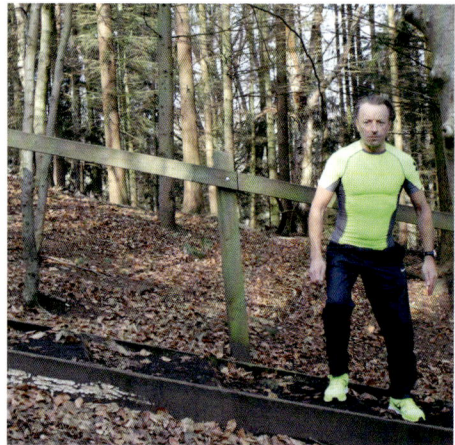
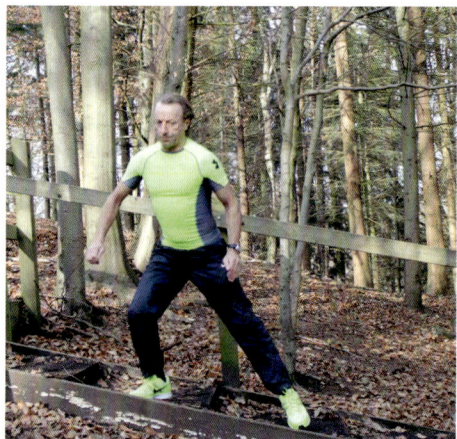

INSTRUCTIONS

- Start with your left side facing the stairs and your left foot on the first step.
- Push down hard on the right foot and take that to the first step and your left foot to the second step.
- Continue this until you reach your marker, and then walk back down the stairs.
- Turn around and now lead with your other foot.
- Repeat this routine 3 times.

EXERCISE 2: SPEED RUNS

Speed runs are as simple as they sound, and they are a great cardio blast for your fitness. They not only increase your heart health but also your lung function and speed.

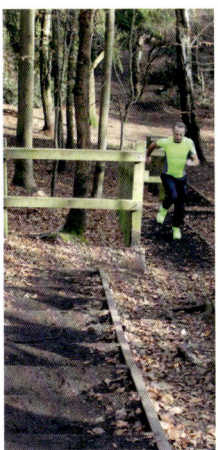 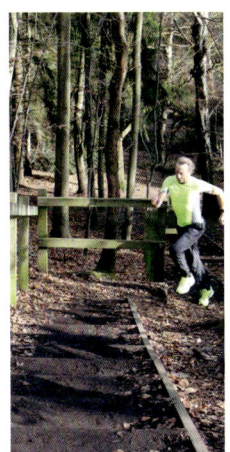 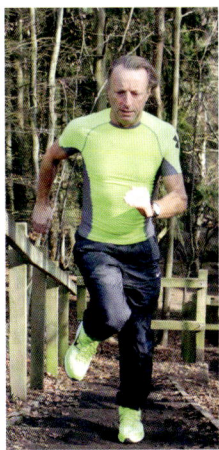 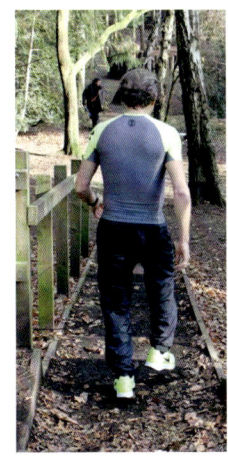 

INSTRUCTIONS
- Using the stair markers placed in the previous exercise, run as fast as you can using your full power and making good use of high knees and coordination to get you to the top in the shortest possible time.
- Slowly walk back down whilst composing yourself.
- Repeat this routine 3 times.

TIPS
- Make sure you have some water on hand to hydrate yourself.
- This is a high-intensity run so make sure you have good footing to avoid tripping.
- If, at any time, you feel any pain or discomfort, then stop.

EXERCISE 3: HOP STAR JUMP

Hopping on two feet is a great plyometric move, which will work your core and quadriceps and improve your balance and stability. This move is tough as you literally engage nearly all of your major muscle groups.

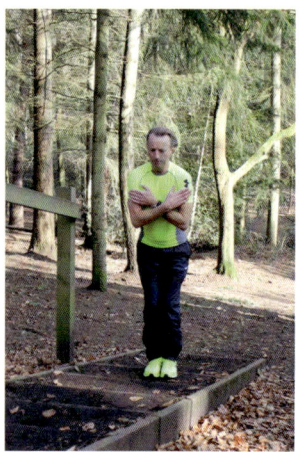 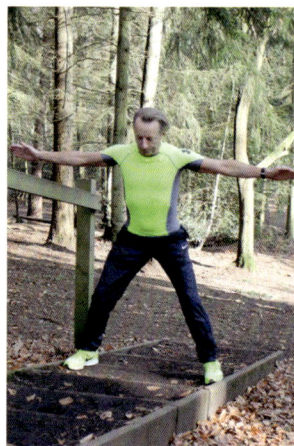 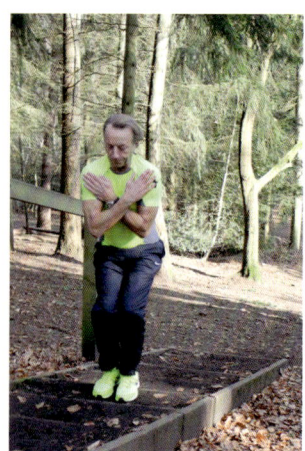

INSTRUCTIONS

- Start with your arms crossed and your feet in a narrow stance with your knees slightly bent.
- Jump up high enough to land on the next step and land in a wide-footed squat position with your arms out to the side like a star jump.
- Jump straight up to the next step, landing back into a narrow stance with your arms crossed again over your chest.
- Keep jumping this sequence up the steps until you reach your marker point.
- Repeat this routine 3 times.

EXERCISE 4: HOP ON ONE FOOT

This exercise will strengthen your lower leg muscles as well as your thighs and glutes, and it will also enhance your balance, stability and core strength.

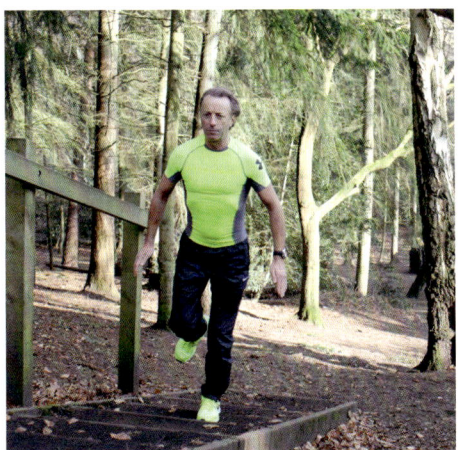
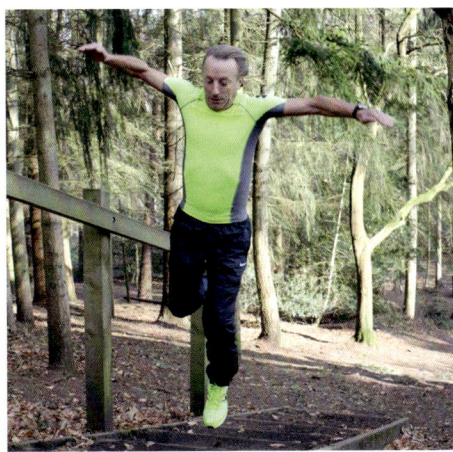

INSTRUCTIONS

- Start by standing on one leg with your core engaged.
- Hop to the first step, keeping good form as it's easy to topple over.
- Continue this movement until you reach your marker, then take your time walking back down.
- Repeat starting with the other leg.
- Repeat this routine 3 times on each leg.

TIP

As you get fitter you can increase the amount of steps you cover.

THE OUTDOOR WORKOUT

EXERCISE 1: BUNNY HOPS

As with many outdoor parks or woods it will never be hard to find a fallen tree. Find one that you will be able to hop over fairly comfortably. This exercise will do wonders for your core strength and upper body.

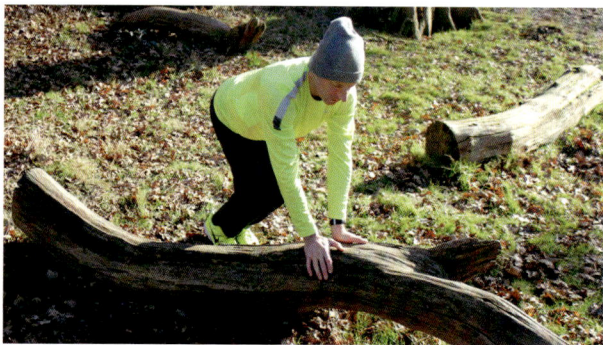

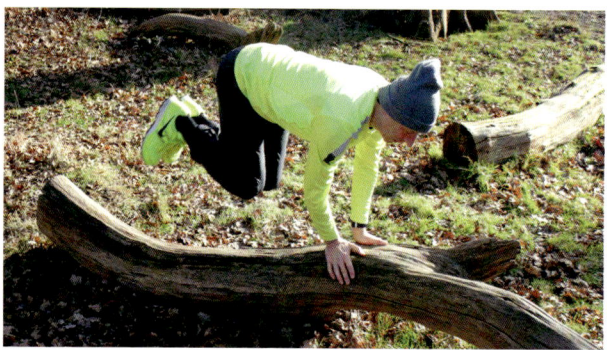

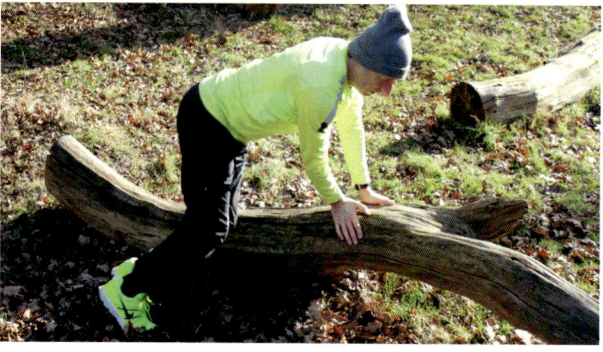

The Ultimate Outdoor Workouts 187

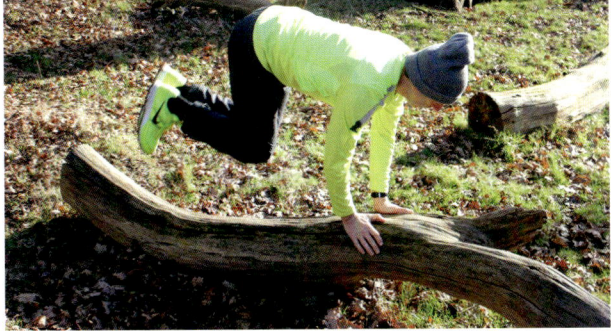

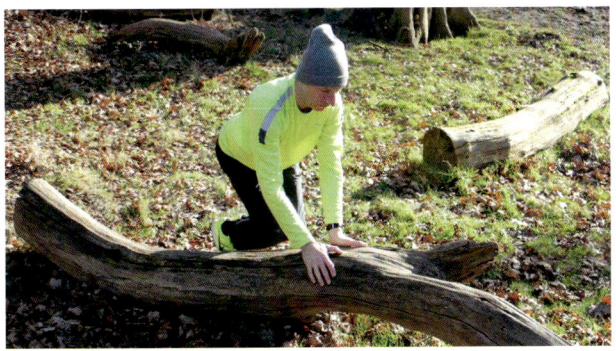

INSTRUCTIONS

- Start by placing your hands firmly on the log, shoulder-width apart. Your legs should be to one side with your knees slightly bent.
- Engage your core and push off from your toes and jump over to the other side keeping your shoulders firmly in front. Keep the momentum going without stopping.
- Repeat this routine doing 3 sets of 20.

EXERCISE 2: STAR JUMP

The star jump is a great way of exercising your legs and your deltoids. It is also a fantastic way of improving your cardio strength. This is a simple exercise and is done in one swift and explosive movement. Your aim is to explode into the star jump continuously for the required amount of reps.

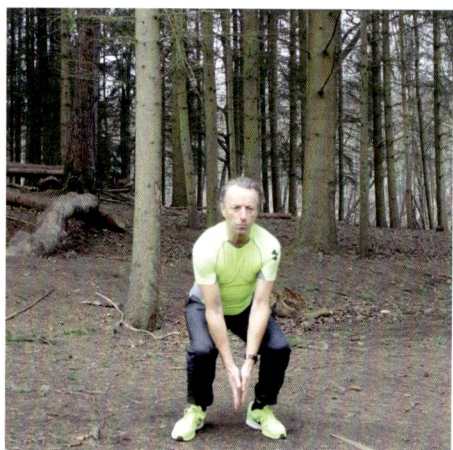 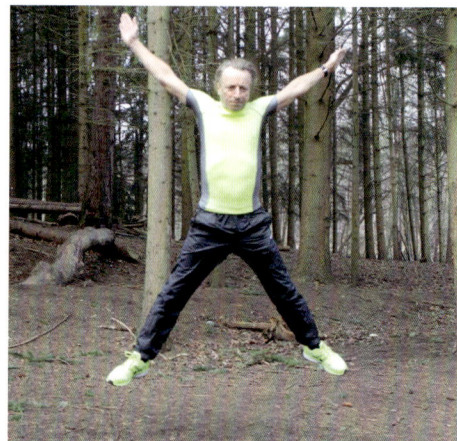

INSTRUCTIONS

- Start by bending your knees into a squat position.
- Explode upwards and outwards, opening your legs wide apart and moving your arms out wide to the side.
- Repeat this routine doing 3 sets of 20.

EXERCISE 3: PULL-UPS

Again, as with many outdoor locations, you are never short of finding something to use to improve your overall body strength. For pull-ups you only need to find a suitable tree with a nice over-hanging branch. This exercise will work your forearms, biceps, triceps and abdominal muscles. Be warned! This is not an easy exercise, as the more weight you have the more you have to pull up. There are two exercises that we can using the tree branch, a straight pull-up and a hanging ab crunch.

VARIATION 1 THE STRAIGHT PULL-UP

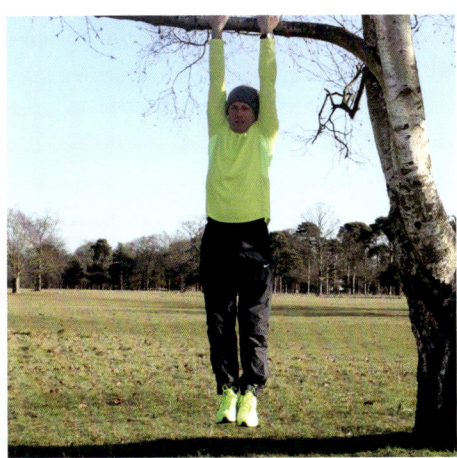
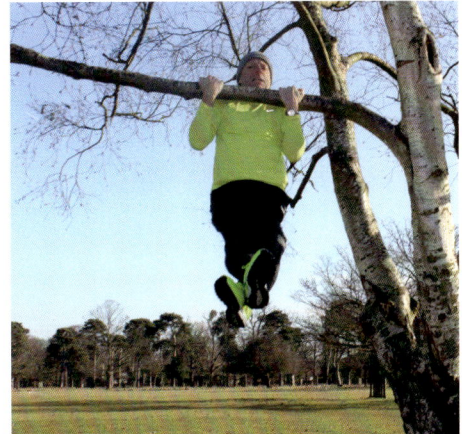

INSTRUCTIONS
- Firmly grip the branch with your hands just past shoulder-width apart and palms facing inwards.
- Fully engage your core muscles, clench your bottom, and try to keep your shoulder blades pinched behind you during this movement.
- Slowly bring your body up so that your chin reaches to the level of the branch. Try to focus on pulling the branch down with your arms and keep the movement controlled without swinging your body.
- Repeat this routine doing 2 sets of 10 pull-ups.

VARIATION 2: THE VERTICAL AB CRUNCH

This vertical ab exercise works the lower part of your abs as you use all the strength to pull your legs up. This exercise is tough but you will quickly notice that the more often you do it the stronger your abs become.

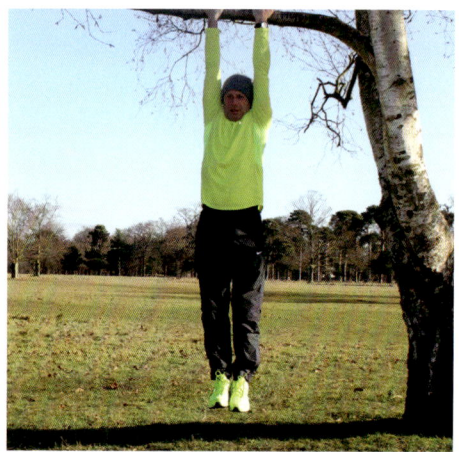 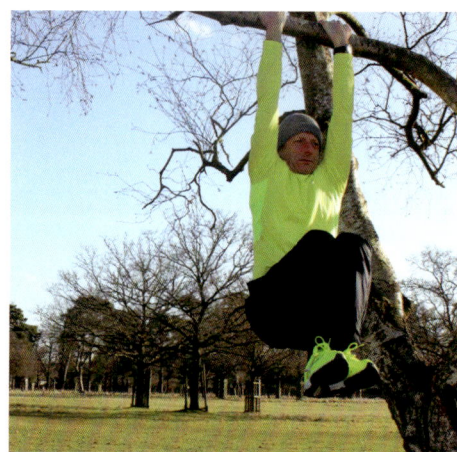

INSTRUCTIONS

- Take a firm grip of your branch with your palms facing you, engage your core muscles, and keep your feet together.
- Raise your knees to your chest in a slow yet fluid movement without swinging your body.
- Hold your knees into your chest for one second and then slowly back to the starting position.
- Repeat this routine 2 sets of 10 crunches.

EXERCISE 4: DECLINE PRESS-UP

A decline press-up is the same movement as the standard press-up, but in this move your body is in an angled position with your feet elevated above your hands. This is more challenging than the standard press-up as you now have more weight over your hands and, as a result, more weight to push up than when your feet are at the same level as your hands. This exercise can be done anywhere outside. The best equipment you can use is a park bench, but you may need to start with a lower height and gradually increase as you get stronger.

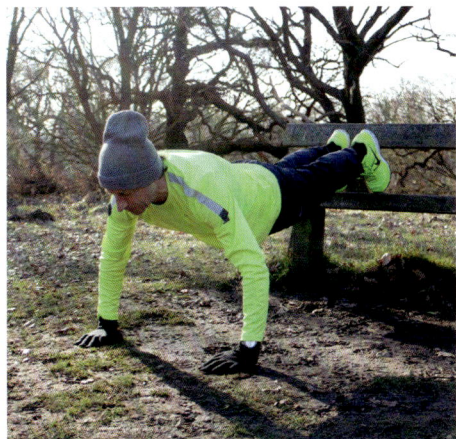
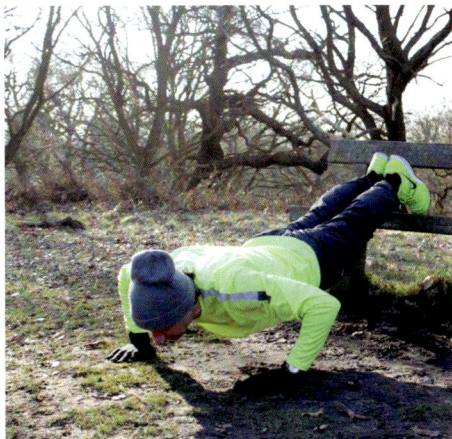

INSTRUCTIONS

- Find a bench or similar object to elevate your feet.
- Keep your hands just past shoulder-width apart and keep a straight line from your ankles to your shoulders. Try not to let your hips drop or rise during this movement.
- With good controlled form, slowly drop down just like a standard press-up and continue back to the starting position.
- Repeat this routine doing 2 sets of 10.

EXERCISE 5: THE LOG JUMP

This high-impact move is a multi-tasker as it not only builds lower body strength but also increases your cardiovascular fitness. This exercise will certainly get the heart pumping.

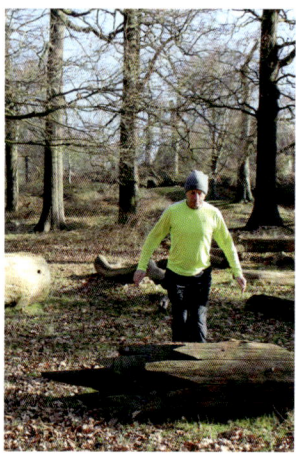
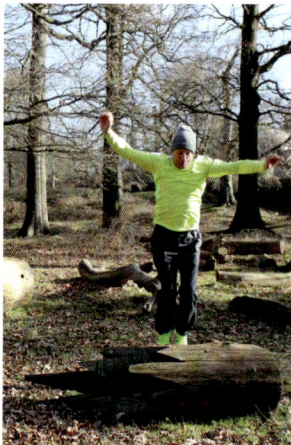
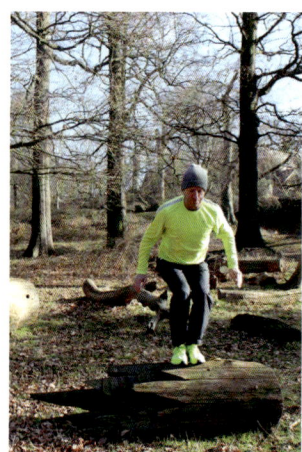

INSTRUCTIONS

- Check the log is solid and stable and make sure the height is not too high. Be sure the log has a good landing area and is not too slippery. The ground should be even and there should be nothing you can slip or twist your ankle on.
- Start by facing the log with your feet hip-width apart, your knees slightly bent, and arms out to your sides.
- Bend your knees more and jump up, aiming to land softly on the log.
- Hold for a second and then jump back down. Keep repeating this move without stopping.
- Repeat this routine doing 2 sets of 12.

TIP

To increase your strength and range of movement, try a higher log to jump up to.

EXERCISE 6: INCLINE PRESS-UP

The incline press-up builds and defines your arms, chest and shoulders. This exercise also fully engages your core muscles for stability.

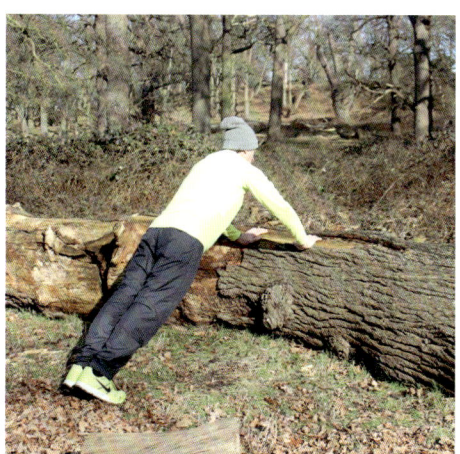
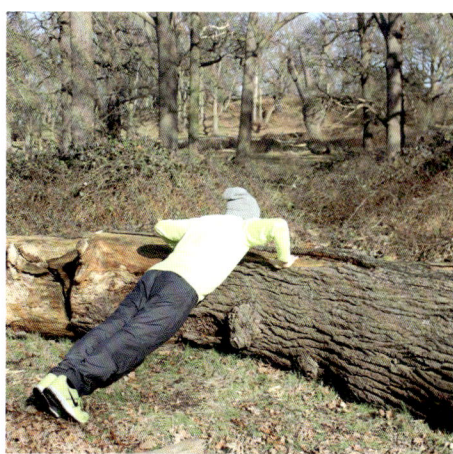
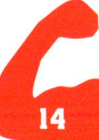

INSTRUCTIONS

- Start by standing a body-length away from the log.
- Gently lean into the log and get yourself into the start of the press-up position with your feet together.
- Ensure your hips are dropped low and that there is a straight line from your heels to your head. Your hands should be wider than shoulder-width apart and your fingers pointing forwards.
- Pull in your tummy muscles and then slowly lower your body down towards the log.
- Hold for a second then slowly push back up.
- Repeat this routine doing 2 sets of 20.

EXERCISE 7: INCLINE STAR PLANK

This exercise engages your waist muscles and helps you with upper body flexibility. Many people find that being stuck on a computer causes them to suffer from back problems; this exercise is great at opening up the chest and preventing back problems.

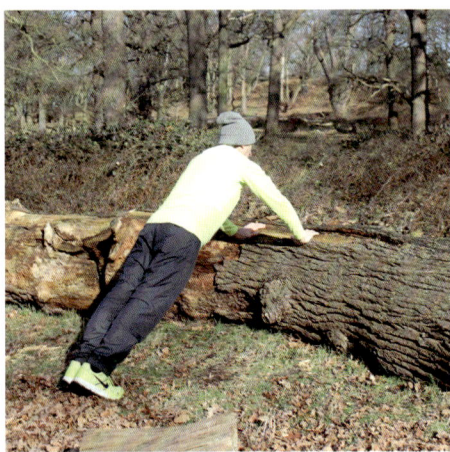
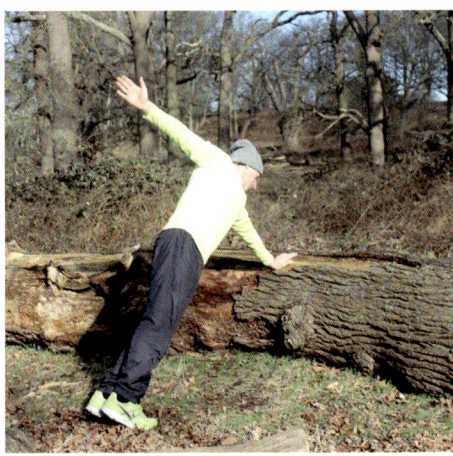

INSTRUCTIONS

- Stand a body-length away from the log.
- Now gently lean into the log and get yourself into the start of the press-up position with your feet together.
- Ensure your hips are dropped low and your body is in a straight line. Keep your hands shoulder-width apart.
- Engage your abdominals, slowly twist your shoulder, and extend one arm out and up as far as you can.
- Hold for a second, then lower back to the start position and repeat on the other arm.
- Repeat this routine doing 2 sets of 20.

The Ultimate Outdoor Workouts   195

Outdoor fitness makes you feel alive and energised. It should be fun and enjoyable as nature has the best gym you can find.

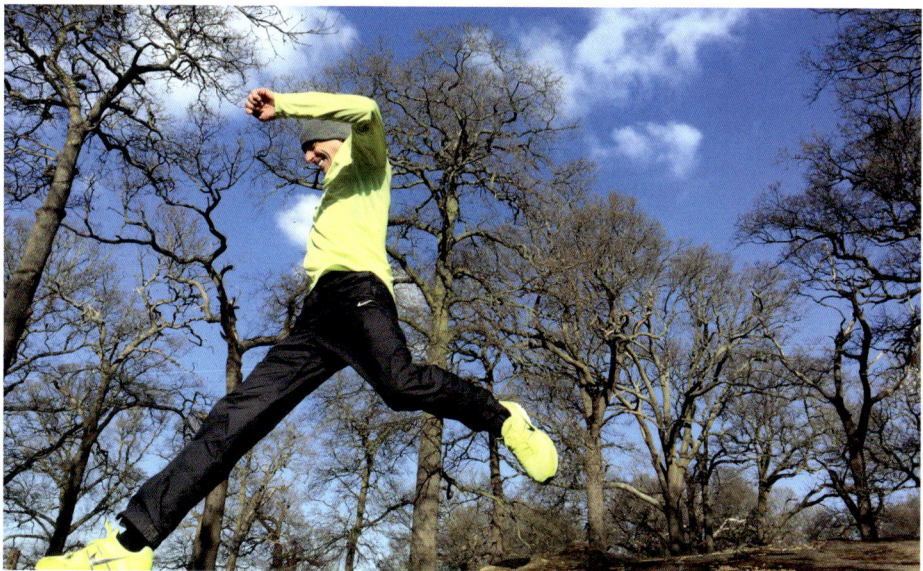

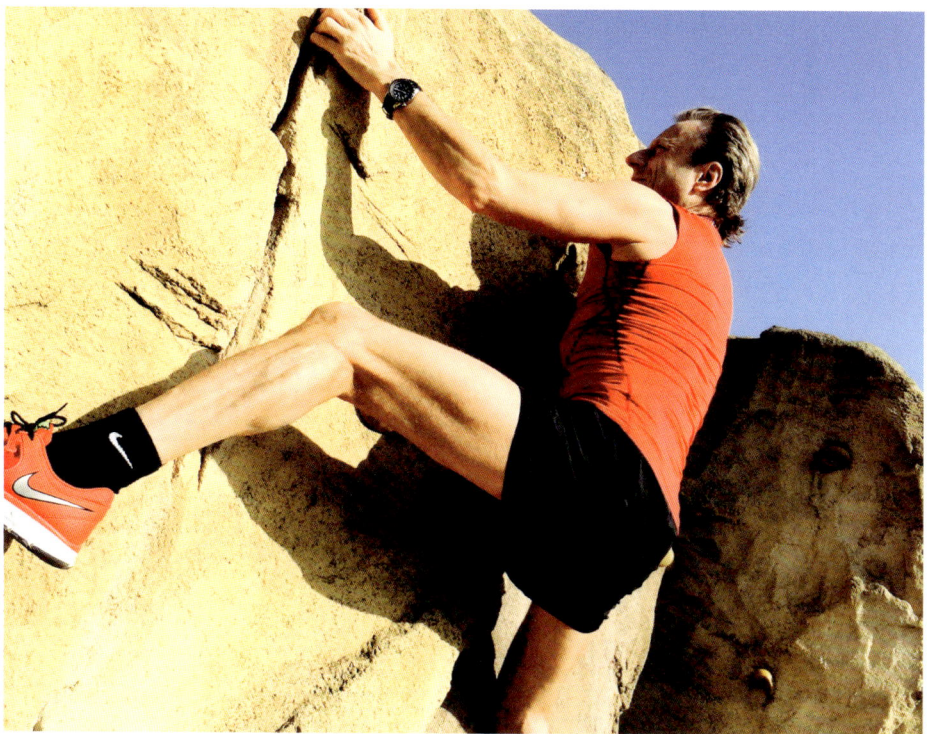

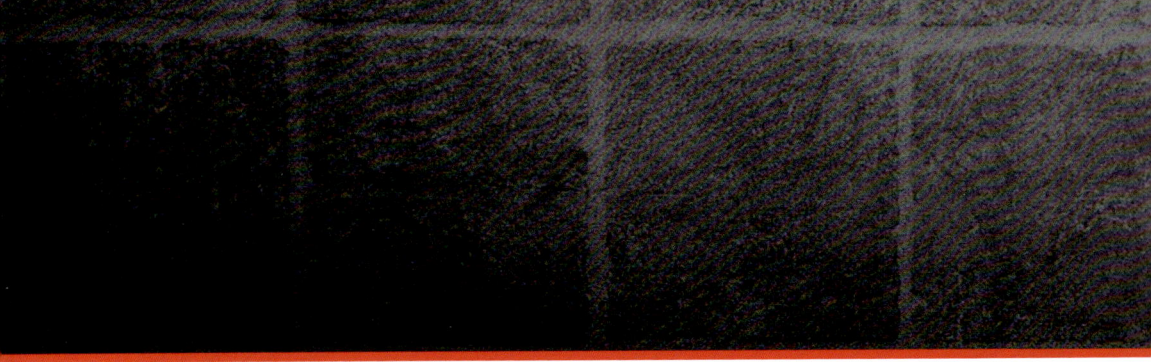

15 REPAIRING YOUR BODY

FOAM ROLLER

Due to the heavy physical demands you are now putting on your body we need to look at ways of aiding the recovery process. The first thing that springs to mind is a massage; research shows that a massage can reduce tension, stiffness and soreness by up to 40%. However, having a massage can be expensive and is not for everyone.

One of the best investments you can make, and at a small price, is a foam roller. A foam roller is a cylindrical piece of hard cell foam. It is used for self-massage by applying it to parts of your body. Using your bodyweight to roll various parts of your body over the foam roller will improve your circulation, and it can also be used as part of your warm-up. A foam roller can play an important part in speeding up your recover after exercising as it breaks down the knots that begin to limit your range of motion and interfere with your running form. It will also decrease your risk of injury.

GETTING STARTED

To use the foam roller correctly, simply use your bodyweight to roll gently over it. You will find that some areas will hurt so if this is the case just support your bodyweight elsewhere by using your arms. As your muscles become more relaxed then you can add more weight. This can be a painful experience and you may initially feel tender or bruised so only work within your pain threshold. When you first start using the roller only complete the rolling sessions every other day, and for no longer than 10 minutes each time.

Just like a sports massage it is important to drink plenty of water before and afterwards to flush away any unwanted toxins.

Focus on areas that are tight or have a reduced range of motion and if you find a particularly painful point try to hold that position until the area softens.

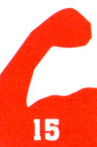

EXERCISE 1: THE GLUTES

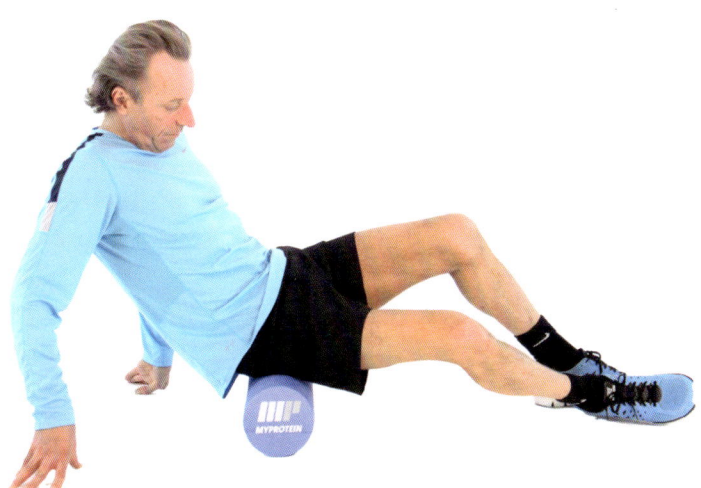

The glutes do a lot of work when you are running and this is an area which will require some attention. Sit on the centre of the foam roller with one leg crossed to the opposite knee. Place both hands on the floor behind you to support your upper body. Gently roll the glute of your bent leg. Now switch leg positions and roll the opposite glute.

EXERCISE 2: THE CALVES

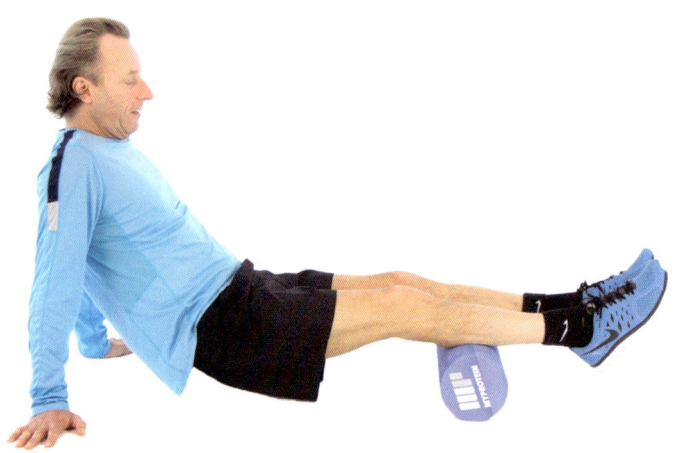

Sit on the floor with your legs straight out, keeping your hands behind you to support your bodyweight. Position the foam roller under your calves and slowly roll your legs up and down from your ankles to your knees, paying particular attention to any stiff and sensitive areas.

EXERCISE 3: THE HAMSTRINGS

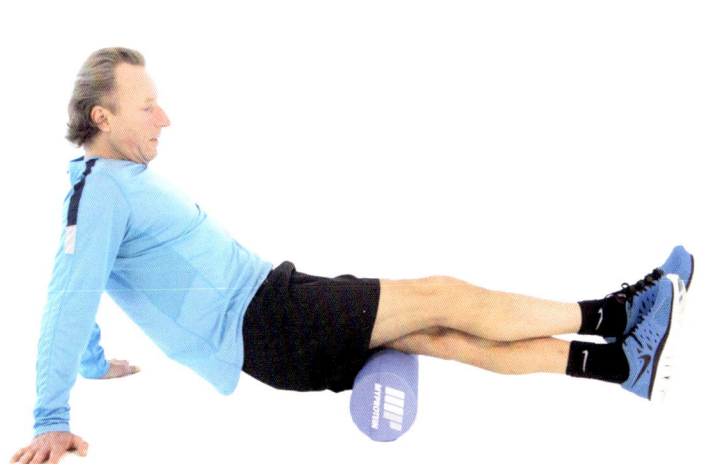

In a sitting position place the roller under your knee with your body weight on the back of your legs and hands behind you. Gently roll from the knees to the buttocks. If you need to increase pressure then roll one leg at a time, turning your leg in and out as you go along.

EXERCISE 4: THE ILIOTIBIAL BAND (IT BAND)

The IT band is the muscle that runs from your hip down to your knee and this is one of the muscles that gets very tight after running.

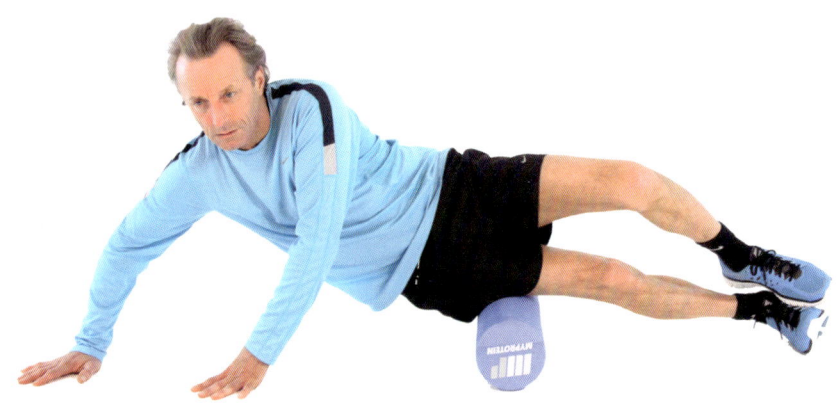

Lie on your side with the roller near your hip and support your upper body on one elbow and forearm. Rest your other leg on the floor. Gently roll yourself along your outer thigh. You can increase the pressure by placing your top leg over your bottom leg.

NOTE

This exercise will test your pain threshold!

EXERCISE 5: THE QUADRICEPS

Lie face down with the roller placed under both thighs. Support yourself on your elbows and forearms, keeping your abs and back muscles slightly flexed to stabilise your spine. Use your bodyweight to roll forward and backward along the front of the thighs, keeping relaxed throughout the movement.

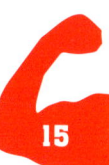

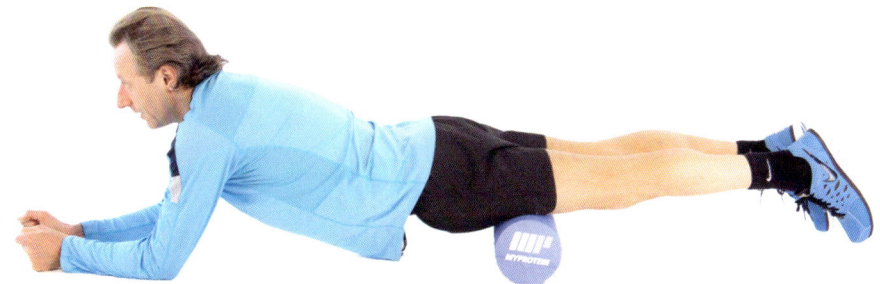

EXERCISE 6: THE BACK

Sit on the floor and place the roller on the lower part of your back. Have your arms out and resting behind you to keep your balance. Engage your abs and slowly bend your knees to move the roller up your back. Take this just to the shoulder blades and back down again.

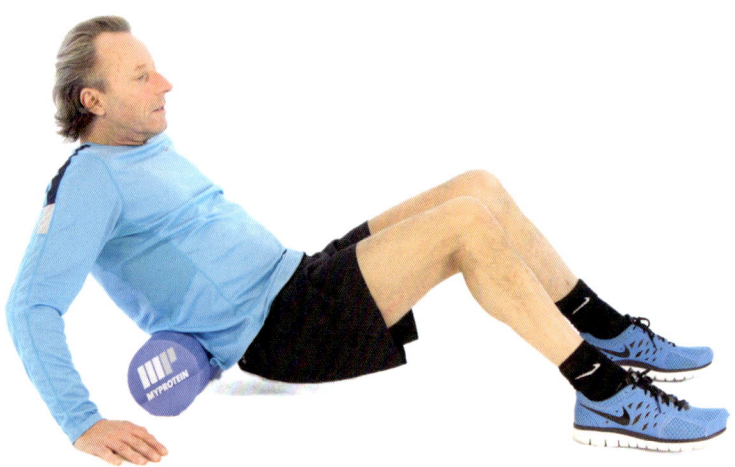

IF YOU SHOULD INJURE YOURSELF

Injury can be common for some people, especially when you push your body to the extreme and ask too much from it. Should you injure yourself when you are running or exercising the most important thing you can do is to stop immediately! You need to make a rough assessment of your injury and look for any signs of sprains, inflammation, bruising or swelling. If you have any of these signs then it is highly recommended to apply ice to the point of injury straight away.

Ice therapy is commonly used in many sporting injuries. When we injure ourselves an increase in blood flow to that area is the body's way of self-healing. This rush of fluid compresses the nerves which ultimately causes the painful swelling. If the swelling isn't controlled it can damage tissues further and therefore needs to be reduced.

Applying a sports pack will:

- Reduce bleeding into the tissues
- Prevent or reduce swelling (inflammation)
- Reduce muscle pain and spasm
- Reduce pain by numbing the area and by limiting the effects of swelling

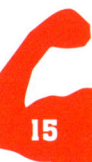

On a very few occasions during my training I have had a slight injury. The best product I have found as a simple yet effective way to repair my injury is the Therapearl sports pack, available at www.therapearl.com.

This amazing product came highly recommended from my running club and is widely used amongst many long-distance runners. The product helps reduce the swelling and prevents the same area from becoming stiff by reducing excess tissue fluid that gathers as a result of injury. Whether it's a torn ligament, bruising or sore muscles, sports packs are great products to use. Simply pop one in the freezer and when you are ready, apply to the injury. The sports pack molds itself around the injured area and very quickly starts to ease the pain and reduce any swelling. When I am training or doing a long distance run I always take a Therapearl sports pack in my rucksack with me just in case I should pick up an injury.

For the best results you should apply sports therapy for up to 20 minutes.

After any injury it is of the upmost importance to allow enough time for complete recovery. Under no circumstance should you rush back into exercise! As frustrating as it may be, you can end up making an injury worse. If your pain is not easing it is always a good idea to get your injury checked out by a doctor or at a sports injury clinic.

16 KEEP UP THE GOOD WORK

So we have now come to the end of this book. I hope that you have found how easy it is to eat well and to include a wide range of exercises into your busy lifestyle. I still lead a busy life and socialise, but now I do it as a fitter and healthier man. You can turn back the years if you look after your body.

Visit my website at www.mensfitkitchen.com and my other social media channels:

 http://instagram.com/mensfitkitchen

 http://pinterest.com/mensfitkitchen

 http://facebook.com/mensfitkitchen

 http://twitter.com/mensfitkitchen

Keep Up the Good Work

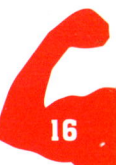

17 ACKNOWLEDGMENTS

Thank you, Lucy Wyndham-Read, for all of your help in getting me this far.

You have inspired and supported to me throughout this journey. I'm proud to call you my friend.

I would also like to thank the very talented and creative director Mr. Mus Rushidi for all his help putting this book together with his unique style, and his beautiful wife Naomi Rushidi for keeping an all-hour help line available to me. Not forgetting the rest of the Rushidi family, thank you to Aidan, Kyla and the very special little princess Erin for making my time at your house so entertaining.

I would also like to thank my sister Christine and brother-in-law Bob for their suggestions and for running their critical eyes over everything I do. I couldn't have done it without you both.

A big thank you to David Lane and Meyer & Meyer for believing in me.

Thank you to all my family, friends and work colleagues who have supported me throughout.

Michael Lloyd, 2015

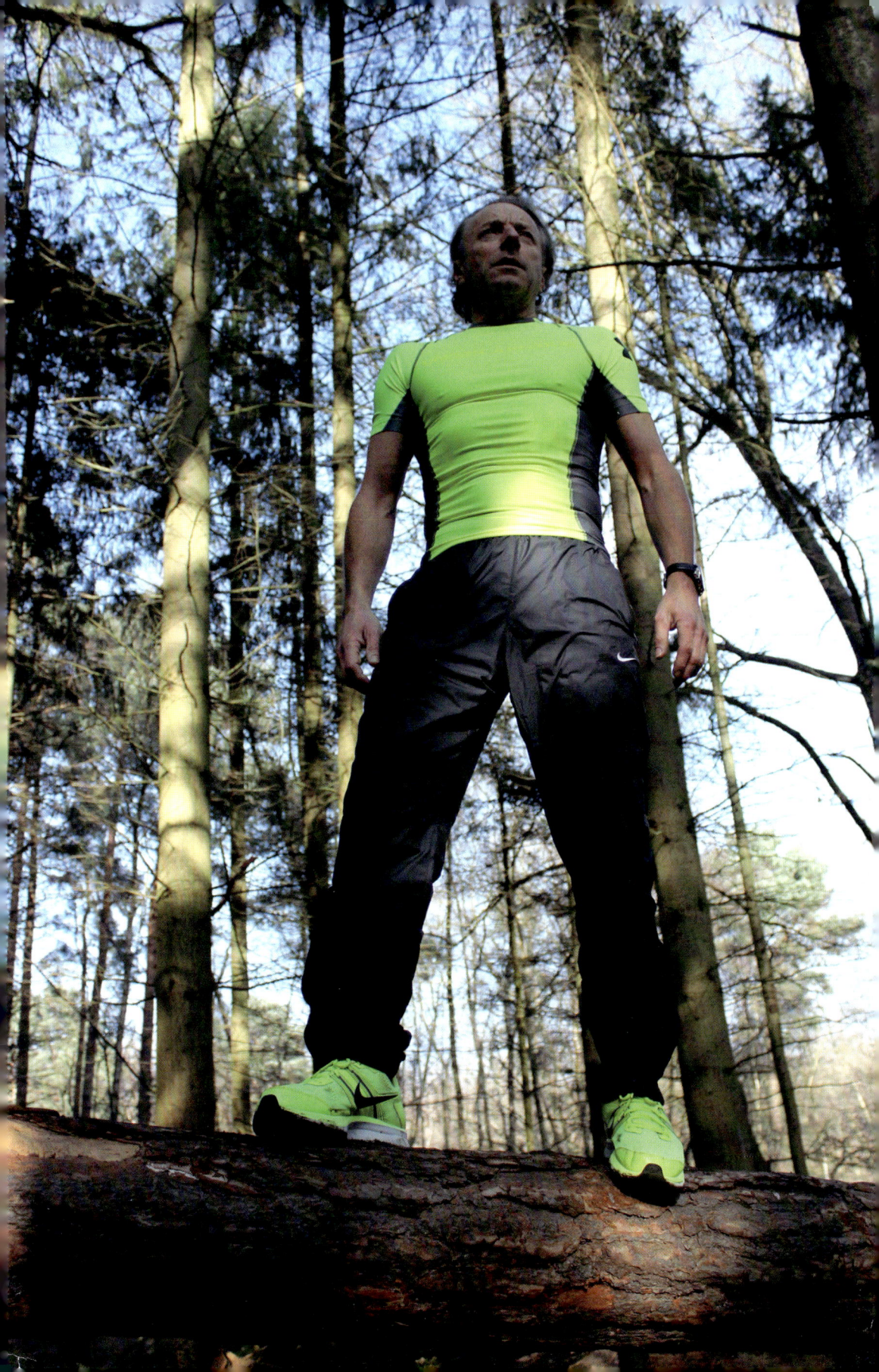

CREDITS

Cover design,
Layout and Typesetting: Sannah Inderest, Aachen

Photographs:

Studio: Axl Stone

Outdoor: Mus Rushidi

Food: Men's Fit Kitchen

© Thinkstock/iStock/Mathieu Boivin: page 35

© Thinkstock/iStock/Metkalova: page: 55

© Thinkstock/Purestock: page 75

Graphics: © Thinkstock/iStock/Javarman3

© Thinkstock/iStock/Artecop2

© Thinkstock/iStock/Lublubachka

© Thinkstock/iStock/Kanate

Copyediting: Anne Rumery